I0707122

MASTERING THE GAME OF LIFELONG WEIGHT LOSS

STUART KREMPIN

Copyright © 2018 by Stuart Krempin.

ISBN: 9781983245596

All rights reserved. No part of this book may be reproduced, stored, or transmitted by any means–whatever auditory, graphic, mechanical or electronic–without written permission of both publisher and author, except in the case of brief excerpts used in critical articles and reviews. Unauthorized reproduction of any part of this work is illegal and is punishable by law.

CONTENTS

PROLOGUE

At the End of my Ability

The sun revealed itself through a faint blue line stretching from the eastern horizon. I thought I was at the end of my ability. My breath had formed ice on my jacket, and I had just brought back sensation to my right hand after wind-milling it in circles to drive warm blood to the fingertips. I just needed to stop moving for a minute, catch my breath if I could, and take account of the situation.

My friend Jake yelled back to me, "You ok, man? You gonna turn back?"

"I'm going to chill for a while," I replied.

Jake looked down at me from his position further up the snowfield and stared for a moment. He left me to my decisions, wherever they would bring me, and continued on.

We were on Pico de Orizaba, Mexico's highest mountain, and I was seriously contemplating turning around. I looked down and shook my head in despair.

"Man...What the hell am I doing?" I said aloud.

The most bizarre feeling overcame me, an exhaustion that permeated so deeply that I felt nauseous. Waves of dizziness passed through me. With my eyes closed, I secured myself onto the steep side of the snowfield by driving my ice axe deep into the ground and sitting by its side.

Ten minutes went by. The only sound was my labored breathing and gusts of air against the ice.

I heard a distant voice, looked up the steep face, and saw Jake yelling to me again, pointing to the west. I hadn't noticed the brilliant sunrise colors. The bottom of the sky was bathed in fiery orange, and our mountain showed its magnitude with a shadow cast over far-off valleys.

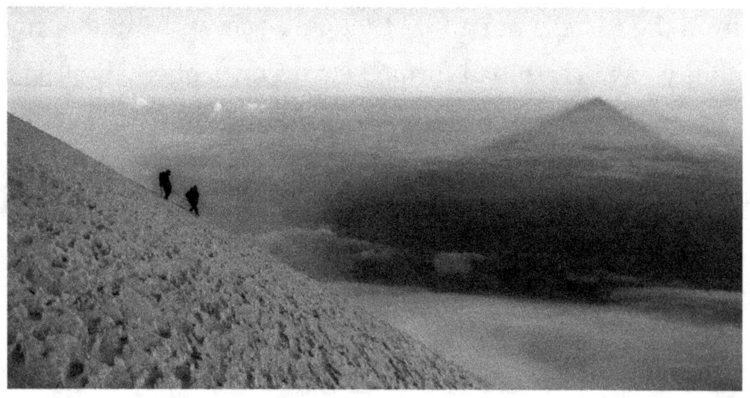

It was too cold. I put on my final layer and stood up on rickety legs. To my surprise, there was no wave of vertigo. I looked up at the summit and continued on.

The day before, we had hired a man to take us to base-camp in his old Jeep Wagoneer. The road was rough, twisting up the mountain to 13,000 feet. The crisp air was already below freezing at this elevation, and we were forced to make the rest of the journey on foot to Orizaba's summit of 18,491 feet. While this expedition was short and could be managed in one long day, I had never been this high, and was, only two days ago, living quite contently at sea level.

After some restless sleep, my alarm woke me up at midnight. Basecamp was already a flurry of activity at this hour, and under normal circumstances, I would be a groggy mess. However, I was quite the opposite, full of energy and ready for a warm meal with my crew who had assembled in one of the makeshift concrete structures scattered near the base of the mountain.

The morning had started like many do in the mountains; we agreed to wake in the wee hours of the night and head off in the dark. It's an eerie endeavor waking up in a rugged and unfamiliar place where darkness veils our concept of distance.

We looked up to the summit, or where we thought it may be, and saw the twinkle of headlamps in the distance resembling something between slowly moving stars and ghostlike specters. These were the parties who decided to beat the crowd and leave earlier than us.

Most acclimatization plans suggest a much more gradual exposure to the higher altitudes. I, however, shrugged the recommendations off, much to the dismay of an inquiring physician who was eating with a group nearby.

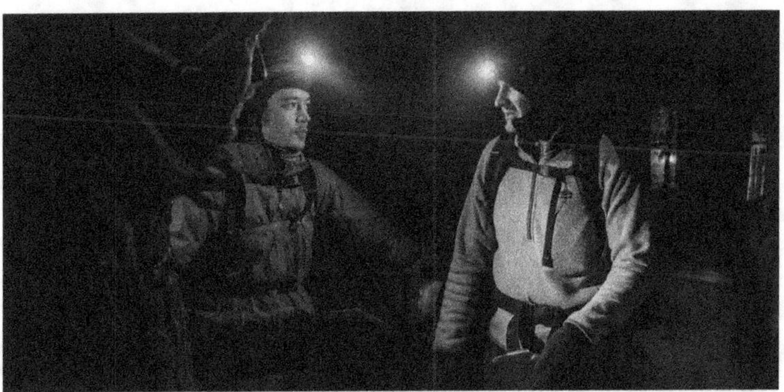

"What mountains have you climbed?" the physician asked us. Jake replied with an impressive list which included multiple climbs of Mount Rainier in Washington as well as some scattered peaks throughout the Cascades north of there. They looked over at me.

"I've been up Rainier once. Almost a vertical mile less than this pretty little dormant volcano. That's about it I guess," I limply retorted with a nervous giggle. The group had a moment of silence in my honor.

"Well, if you start to really lose it, I pray that you have the common sense to turn back," said the doctor with a smile of his own.

I was hoping he wasn't going to have to drag my ass off the mountain with the help of my friend, but inexperienced as I was, there was an underlying confidence I had about myself. I'd soon find out if it was justified.

We ate with determination and marched off similarly. Walking in a single-file line, the jagged cliffs and boulder-strewn mountainside were obscured. We kept our eyes on the headlamp-lit ground while trying not to look at the distant lights of other climbers above us. The objective was one step in front of the next.

"Just keep walking, and stop worrying yourself with the big picture," I told myself. I'd grown accustomed to silencing the nagging voice in the back of my mind over the years. That skill would serve me well today.

Losing Sight

As I climbed, I recalled the first time I played in the snow as a child. It was on Mount Wilson, where, at its summit, the city of Los Angeles is faintly visible in the distance. It was only a melted slush by the time I saw the snow, but there was still a sense that magical things were found in these hard-to-reach places.

There was no way the child version of me could fathom navigating a trip to Mount Wilson on my own, but luckily I had a dad who was willing to make the winding drive to the top. The world looked very small below, complex but also more peaceful in a way. We would sit atop the mountain and stare out at the urban sprawl below us in silence.

A lot of the best memories I accumulated as a kid were the ones away from the city. This included hiking, camping, and mountain biking in unfamiliar places, in which I found an exciting sense of exploration and discovery.

The outdoors fueled my imagination. I was a daydreamer in school, and, to this day, often find myself taking a mental journey through past exploits.

The real-world is a place filled with political parties, bills, taxes, multiple-choice tests, achy backs, Netflix, and takeout. After many years, I lost sight of the world of exploration and adventure as the insidious effects of the 'real-world' over-came my reality.

My parents were also overcome by this 'real-world,' fighting over bills and threatening divorce multiple times. It seemed that the happiest family moments were somewhere between the second and third plate at the Silver Bullet Casino steak night buffet. Life was often a bummer, and food became medicine.

Healthy eating was not on my radar as a kid. Except for infrequent outdoor adventures, I stayed inside, playing Super Nintendo and watching television. Inactivity and poor diet choices became the standard, and I blew up. By the fifth grade, I took the throne as the heaviest kid in class and was easily gassed with low-impact playground games.

This continued for some time, through my teens and most of my twenties. I became really sad, and yet I used the one thing that was slowly killing me as a medication: food. I realize now the problem I had was addiction. I was addicted to the rush of feel-good hormones a plate of junk food gave me.

I was deep in my addiction by the time I went to college and became really unhealthy. When I dropped out of college, things got worse.

> **Food addiction:** Using food as an emotional stabilizer and a coping mechanism. It is self-propagating, fueled by the feel-good hormones and sense of fulfillment satiety gives you. Food addiction brings a continuous preoccupation with eating and is driven from a more instinctual and subconscious area of the mind. It's normal to think about food, but those who've entered the realm of addiction have an unnatural preoccupation with thoughts about it and participate in activities such as 'grazing' and binge-eating.

During these college years, I remember sitting in the blood donation center with a technician listening to my heart with a confused look on her face. After a few minutes spent verifying her findings, she looked up to me and said I'd better go see a doctor.

"Your heart is skipping over ten beats a minute," she said with concern. She checked my blood pressure, which produced a reading you'd expect to see in a woman giving birth. If it hadn't been for my attempt to be a good samaritan, I would have never realized my desperate health state.

When I did see my family doctor, it was no surprise when he prescribed a diet and some blood pressure medicine. I was sick and I needed to kick my food addiction. I returned year after year with no success, and he was less than impressed. I couldn't bring myself to continue reporting my failure, so I stopped going. The guilt trip I was receiving from my doctor, as well as myself, couldn't have been less helpful.

Those early days were tough, yet it was through those struggles that I was able to forge myself anew. I always had hope things would improve, but hope is not the path, it's just the compass. I never knew that, eventually, walking on the right path would bring me to the adventurous life the kid-version of me spent so much time dreaming about.

The Summit

As I looked towards the summit of Orizaba, I thought about all that I had been through to get here, The instincts developed through years of hardship re-surfaced.

I said to myself, "one step at a time," and took that step, then some breaths, and another step. There was a cadence in my march up the mountain, matched easily with my breathing, never so fast that I lost the rhythm. If the step was large, I took some time with more breathing. I finally regained my composure and walked ahead with conviction.

The sun was rejuvenating. I looked up often towards the horizon and its pastel wonder. That's when the smile came, a small signal that I was doing ok. I repeated this mantra in my mind, maybe a hundred times or more while walking: "You got this, Stuart, you got this. Nice and easy, no problem."

My climbing partner had dusted me, I was in the back and had already been passed by another team. In the back of my mind, my ego was cringing, but I gave myself some encouragement. That's what I really needed as I was nearing the top, walking deeper into exhaustion than ever before.

It's as if it were just a blink, after the switch in mindset. Before that, time was slow and each step was a struggle, but after, time flew until I walked on the summit and met up with friends who were taking in the full warmth of the sun now beaming brightly. It felt amazing; I too was beaming.

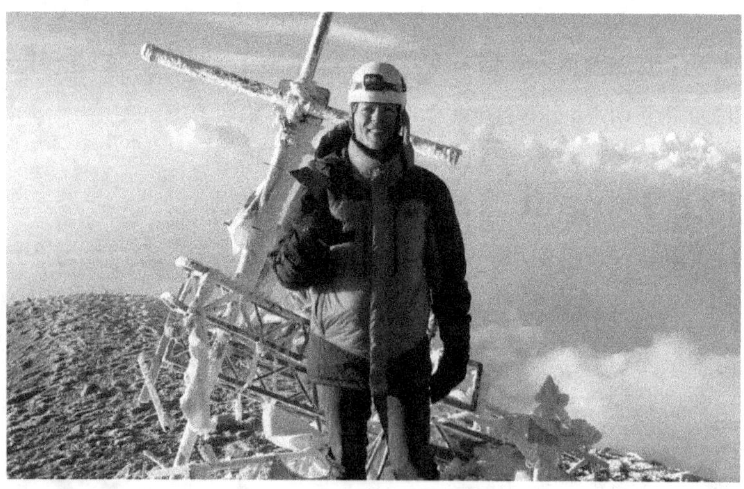

"Halfway done," Jake said with a sigh.

"At least we're done with the hard half!" I replied.

There was something magical found at the top of Orizaba when I eventually lumbered off the summit. Big, scary, and far off, this goal had been a distant horizon. And now I was walking back down the mountain, having met a momentous challenge. I had spent so much time working it up in my mind, and then just like that, *poof*, I headed back to base-camp. It took some time for reality to catch up.

It's fun, and almost a safe feeling to have that impossible goal looming out of reach. After achieving this goal, every-thing gets complicated again. It's a feeling that you can't really prepare for.

There was a shockwave that passed through my body, mimicking the same feeling I obtained when I finally real-ized my original weight loss goal many years earlier. Life had been happening really fast since then. My body trans-formation had become a stepping stone that eventually led me to the summit of Mexico's highest mountain. If that's where the story ended, that'd be awesome, but things kept getting better.

The Inner Transformation

This book is not about what comes after your transformation, because that part depends on the extent of your imagination. We start much earlier, for those who may be at the beginning of their journey (perhaps again) wondering what it'll take to merge into the fast lane and finally succeed. While, yes, this is about **Mastering the Game of Lifelong Weight Loss**, it's really about mastering one's self.

"It's the mind that really creates the body, it is the mind that makes you really work the 4 or 5 hours a day. It's the mind that visualizes what the body is to look like as the finished product."

ARNOLD SCHWARZENEGGER

Before climbing a single mountain, I had to pursue mastery of myself (which is always a work in progress). I was absolutely lost, but my dream was to escape a body that I felt had cursed me. While there are much worse fates than being obese, I had associated nearly all of my stunted progress in life to this runaway weight issue.

I journeyed in a very inefficient course, zigging and zagging to every hack, habit, and system I could find. My goal was effective fat loss that lasted, not breakneck weight-loss speed records.

Truth be told, I wasted a lot of time and energy on many detours. Now, I'd like to help others take a more direct route.

The powerful lessons below took me decades to learn, and are the backbone of this book. They have been obtained through real-world trial and error, and are practical and effective.

What Will You Learn from this Book?

- How to craft picture-perfect goals and action plans.
- How to reprogram your habits.

- The right mentality with food and how to defeat weight loss plateaus.
- How to find your place within fitness.
- How to become a motivational guru.
- How to visualize your ideal future.
- How to create the ideal environment for growth.
- How to follow the path of positive thinking.

As a byproduct of mastering myself, the external changes have been staggering. My transformation was accomplished with no drugs, surgery, or personal trainer. The tactic I employed was self-empowerment through seeking out the right kind of information and acting on it.

Below, you can see images that represent both my personal rock bottom and the achievement of my original weight loss goal. Within these pages is everything it took for me to get there.

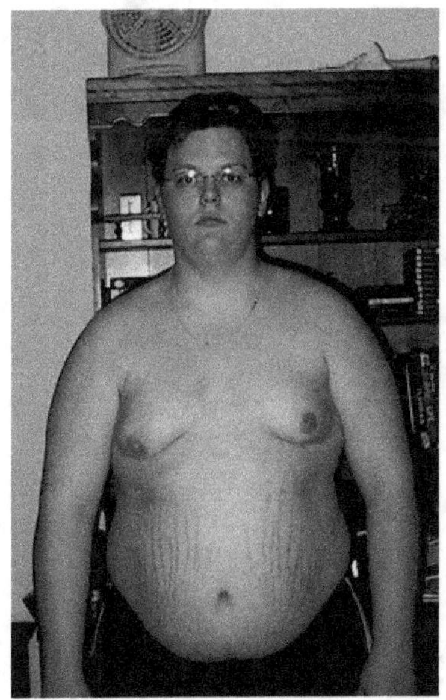
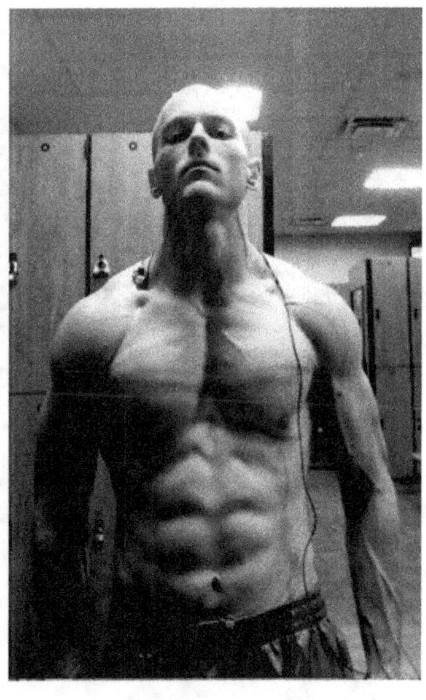

These outward changes helped me to believe in my own value. We all have value deep within us. For some, however, it takes a special effort to realize it.

When you get what you want in your struggles for pelf,
And the world makes you King for a day,
Then go to a mirror and look at yourself,
And see what that guy has to say.

For it isn't your Father, or Mother, or Wife
Who judgment upon you must pass.
The fellow whose verdict counts most in your life
Is the guy staring back from the glass.

You may be like Jack Horner and "chisel" a plum,
And think you're a wonderful guy,
But the man in the glass says you're only a bum
If you can't look him straight in the eye.

He's the fellow to please, never mind all the rest
For he's with you clear to the end
And you've passed your most dangerous, difficult test
If the guy in the glass is your friend.

You can fool the whole world down the pathway of years,
And get pats on the back as you pass,
But your final reward will be heartache and tears
If you've cheated the man in the glass.

DALE WIMBROW, THE GUY IN THE GLASS

THE ADVENTURE BEGINS

What was the event that sparked the push for change? I'm often asked this question, and I can't trace it back to one thing. My issues became so toxic to me that a breaking point was inevitable. Some of them included:

- Very real effects on my health, including high blood pressure, heart arrhythmias, knee joint damage, and posture changes from the weight of my stomach pulling my spine out of alignment.
- Feeling socially oppressed and way too fearful of events that involved any form of water (pool, beach, inner tubing).
- Bottomed-out self-confidence, and a belief that I had zero control of my circumstances.
- Having to get off the rollercoaster and walk away after being unable to close the waist bar.
- Blowing out every pair of pants I have ever owned as I was bending over to pick something up, usually in public with no change of clothes nearby.
- Feeling unworthy of a lot of things just because I was unhappy with myself.
- Needing a helicopter rescue out of a canyon in California after clumsily breaking my leg.

Unfortunately, I let it get to a point where my health was genuinely affected. Some of us really need to hit rock bottom before we're able to change. I was definitely there.

You've undoubtedly heard someone mention while diving into some grease-fest, "hey, I don't want to live until I'm 100 years old anyways."

I can understand and appreciate the desire to live life to the fullest, but oftentimes these people don't realize the outcome of this lifestyle as I do, having the vantage point of working in healthcare.

I'm sure these people who don't want to reach 100 also didn't associate living out the last half of their lives worried about their runaway health problems, including frequent visits to the hospital, sometimes even ER visits, and 911 calls. But that's how it goes when you "live life to the fullest" in that way. That's the future I desperately wanted to avoid.

What will be your breaking point? Will you let things get so bad that you've dug yourself into a deep well?

Please don't wait until you have significant health issues. But if that's the case already, many of your woes are reversible, so don't waste another second. I hope you never let it get to that point though.

> "Every adversity, every failure, every heartache carries with it the seed of an equal or greater benefit."
>
> NAPOLEON HILL, "THINK AND GROW RICH"

After hitting rock bottom, I stumbled upon an internet community of individuals who were facing the same health struggles as I was. One thing really stuck with me—lots were winning the battle of transforming themselves. After I read one success story after another, I truly started to believe it could happen to me.

Belief is important. You *must* believe that you can win the battle. Research shows that "It was belief itself that made the difference. Once people learned how to believe in something, that skill started spilling over to other parts of their lives, until they started believing they could change."[1]

I want you to know it's possible. I want to show you that any average person can really get a redo on their life.

I have transformed myself.
Many others have done it.
YOU can transform yourself too!

The world is full of people conquering their goals and transforming their lives. Difficult as it may be, change is not a fairytale, and realizing this makes believing possible.

Start With a Vision

As a child, you likely looked up to heroes who embodied the ideal virtues of humanity: strong, brave, decisive, and intelligent. You may have thought that if you tried hard enough, you could gain some of these powers, perhaps if you ate enough spinach or did enough sit-ups. As we grow up, however, life can curb our imagination and make those ideas seem childish.

I remember, as a kid, thinking about the man I wanted to become. I remember this man as if he were a real figure, standing tall and confident with the look of satisfaction that an accomplished person has. The fears I suffered in reality were nonexistent in him.

I didn't know at the time, but this was a prelude to my vision. I've found that, through the years, having a strong vision of the person you want to become will act as a compass when you get too comfortable.

During my journey, I imagined this figure looking back and telling past me, "keep pushing, you're not there yet, but every day you're building yourself, one small victory at a time, into an epic human being."

> "What you do is create a vision of who you want to be, and then live into that picture as if it were already true."
>
> ARNOLD SCHWARZENEGGER,
> "TOTAL RECALL: MY UNBELIEVABLY TRUE LIFE STORY"

Beyond the pep talk, progress is only made by taking action. In the coming segments, I'll occasionally provide an action for you to accomplish. To build the person we want to become, we must build from the ground up. In the beginning, we start with your vision.

Transforming takes effort, and keeping track of the bits and pieces of your transformation will be an important part of the process. That's why we all need our own **transformation journal**. I'll identify times that there is important information that would best be written in the transformation journal, by suggesting you **Write It Down**.

To start things off, we can create our Personal Vision. Make it visual, like a photograph in your mind. Then, answer these five questions in a statement about your future self.

- What are your virtues?
- What do you look like?
- What will you accomplish?
- What is your life like?
- What are some things this future person would say to your current self?

This is highly personal. This is about you. There's no right or wrong way to do this exercise, but please, make sure that you do it. Your emotions can bring about power. The fire from within will drive you to pursue this vision of yourself and your life. If you create that dominant emotional connection with your vision, you will be invested in the outcome. The ability to lead the excellent life you envision, and be the person you've imagined, is truly within reach of each and every one of us.

Develop Goals

"If you aim at nothing you will hit it every time."

ZIG ZIGLAR, AMERICAN MOTIVATIONAL SPEAKER AND AUTHOR

It's not enough to have lofty ideas of the things you want to accomplish. In the previous section, we used some visualization techniques to dream up the ideal version of us. This was only a rough picture.

Having this picture in your mind may push you to certain levels of progress, but instead of softly laying out an idea of what you want, you must go through the effort of taking it to the next level. By having a properly laid-out goal, you have a definite point to work towards. In this section, I'll describe a specific, tried-and-true methodology for setting goals.

Rewind to the beginning of this year. People that go to the gym regularly, and have been going for a while, know that January can be a disheartening month. You circle the parking area a few times to find a spot, thinking, "pretty busy today, what the heck." You park, go in and realize...

> *"Oh yeah... It's January, the New Year's crowd has arrived."*

The gym is suddenly filled with people all wanting to make positive changes in their lives, and that's great, although sometimes frustrating when you have to wait to jump on a machine. The sad truth about the matter is that the gym will likely be back down to its typical occupancy by February or March at the latest.

While there may be more to the picture than a lack of goals, part of the problem is not having a definite idea of what they intend on accomplishing. It may be ideas such as:

"I'd like to get back into shape," or
"I want to get a flatter tummy,"
or any number of different vague ideas.

When you have no specific plan, it's hard to tell if you're making any real strides towards your vision.

But setting attainable goals is easy, and it helps to use a blueprint. You'll want to make goals that are **specific**, **measurable**, and that have a defined **timeline**.

Specific

When people make goals, they typically leave a lot of information up to the imagination. Having specific goals creates a roadmap that's much more obvious and tangible.

I have always considered Arnold Schwarzenegger to be an inspiration and have spent lots of time reading up on his wisdom. In order to design the future that he wanted for himself, he used very specific goals to direct his actions. Here, he talks about his goal-oriented mind early in his career:

"I always wrote down my goals, like I'd learned to do in the weight-lifting club back in Graz. It wasn't sufficient to just tell myself something like, "My New Year's resolution is to lose twenty pounds and learn better English and read a little bit more." No. That was only a start. Now I had to make it very specific so that all those fine intentions were not just floating around. I would take out index cards and write that I was going to:

- *get twelve more units in college;*
- *earn enough money to save $5,000;*
- *work out five hours a day;*
- *gain seven pounds of solid muscle weight; and*
- *find an apartment building to buy and move into.*

It might seem like I was handcuffing myself by setting such specific goals, but it was actually just the opposite: I found it liberating. Knowing exactly where I wanted to end up freed me totally to improvise how to get there."

You can see that there wasn't much ambiguity about the kinds of things he wanted.

Measurable

When your specific goal is measurable, you're able to see incremental progress and know when it has been achieved.

Let's turn some lofty goals into specific and measurable goals.

- I want to get in shape. ➤ I will run a half marathon.
- I want to see my abs. ➤ I will have 10% body fat.
- I want to eat healthier. ➤ I will cut out french fries and soda from my diet.

Timeline

The last part of making a goal is giving it a timeframe. Sitting on a goal without giving it a timeframe leads to goal stagnation. We want a deadline! Pressure is good because it empowers us to take action.

Give your goals a timeframe, a realistic timeframe, so that you have a way to tackle what you need to do by when. Think of timelines in daily, weekly, monthly, and yearly chunks. You'll be able to know what's realistic after some time in the trenches working through these goals.

Long-term and Short-term Goals

Is it reasonable for a broke college student to have a goal of being a millionaire? In the long-term, absolutely. Is it reasonable for a morbidly obese person to have a goal of competing in a bodybuilding show with 6% body fat? Sure, why the hell not.

Oprah Winfrey said she'd be a millionaire by 32, and ended up being one of the richest women in the world. She once said, "The big secret in life is that there is no big secret. Whatever your goal, you can get there if you're willing to work."

Arnold Schwarzenegger knew what he wanted as well: to be the world's greatest bodybuilder. He worked his butt off to get there, and eventually the title was his, seven times over. There's not much that's unattainable if you're willing to make sacrifices and put in the work.

You can accomplish whatever you want, but long-term goals must be broken down to shorter-term ones. Since common people have accomplished great things, don't fear to dream big. Those big dreams of yours should contain a set of shorter-term goals to break things down. Michael Jordan, the famous American Basketball Player, had this to say about creating more manageable goals to lead up to your monstrous ones.

> "I approach everything step by step...I had always set short-term goals. As I look back, each one of the steps or successes led to the next one. When I got cut from the varsity team as a sophomore in high school, I learned something. I knew I never wanted to feel that bad again....So I set a goal of becoming a starter on the varsity. That's what I focused on all summer. When I worked on my game, that's what I thought about. When it happened, I set another goal, a reasonable, manageable goal that I could realistically achieve if I worked hard enough...I guess I approached it with the end in mind. I knew exactly where I wanted to go, and I focused on getting there. As I reached those goals, they built on one another. I gained a little confidence every time I came through.
>
> ...If [your goal is to become a doctor]... and you're getting Cs in biology then the first thing you have to do is get Bs in biology and then As. You have to perfect the first step and then move on to chemistry or physics.
>
> Take those small steps. Otherwise you're opening yourself up to all kinds of frustration. Where would your confidence come from if the only measure of success was becoming a doctor? If you tried as hard as you could and didn't become a doctor, would that mean your whole life was a failure? Of course not.

All those steps are like pieces of a puzzle. They all come together to form a picture...Not everyone is going to be the greatest...But you can still be considered a success... Step by step, I can't see any other way of accomplishing anything."

MICHAEL JORDAN, "I CAN'T ACCEPT NOT TRYING: MICHAEL JORDAN ON THE PURSUIT OF EXCELLENCE"

By breaking down his epic goals, Jordan made his pathway clear. The truth is that, until I made smaller goals part of my own path, I was putting myself under a great deal of undue stress.

When I was a kid, I thought it would be awesome to be buff and ripped. I grew up with this dream, and every time I saw myself in the mirror, it gave me a painful jolt as reality slapped me in the face. While I enjoyed seeing the fruits of my dedication to better myself, I was often distracted by my daunting goal. It felt so far away that I couldn't see it. Being thin felt conceptual at best, as if it were a physics theory that scientists could only conjecture about. When a weight loss attempt slowed to a halt, I would lose sight of my goal and become lost.

What is sometimes difficult to see in published success stories about amazing people is the "in-between" stuff. All the trials and challenges between the kid and the hero. It wasn't a lightning bolt delivered from Zeus that made this person the hero, it was all the in-between stuff, the day-to-day decisions, the small successes, stacked atop each other.

Ed Viesturs, a famous high-altitude mountaineer, made over 200 ascents of Mount Rainier (4,392 meters) before he tackled any of the fourteen 8,000-meter-and-above mountains.

He eventually became the only American to have summited all of them. If that's all you knew about him, you wouldn't realize that he had already spent countless hours prepping, training, and perfecting his craft. His amazing accomplishment was just a puzzle filled with smaller pieces, and that's exactly how he stayed focused when tackling such impressive intentions.

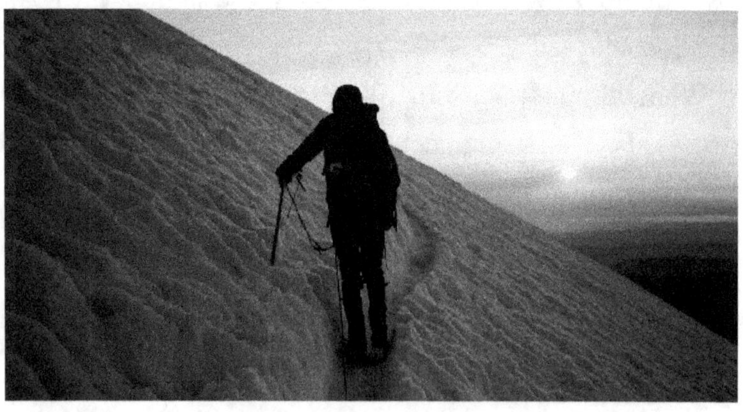

Look at the small pieces, focus on them, in fact. Once you have the right plan, losing that first pound is doable! If you can lose one pound, you can lose two, and three, and so on.

Keep your eyes on the small steps to tackling your transformation. It will put your queasy stomach at ease and remind you not to focus on the far-off summit, but merely to get to the next mile marker in the trek.

This is exactly why it's vital to keep your short-term goals attainable; when they're reasonably sized, they become baby steps.

If you feel anxiety, focus only on that short-term goal. Then, one day, when you look down from your grand summit, you'll see an epic trail made of these small steps.

Goal Setting Summary

The goal system above is an efficient way of producing goals that are effective. The system creates specific and measurable goals with a timeline. Here are a few examples of some solid goals using this blueprint.

- I will lose one pound this week.
- I will walk for two miles, three times this week.
- I will reduce my body fat percentage from ___ to ___ by December.
- I will stop drinking soda for the entire month of ____.

Since this book *is* about transformations, we will talk about ways to help you tackle these goals and the types of goals you'll want.

Consider the following:

- Exercise goals.
- Diet goals.
- Personal measurement goals (weight, belly circumference, etc.).
- Knowledge building goals (reading a health related book).
- Lifestyle goals (quitting smoking, drinking, gambling, or starting to meditate, etc.).
- Fun goals (the bucket list!).

Creating a list of 200 goals at once is a bad idea. Start small with long and short-term goals for just a few things. Then build the list as you check the most important ones off.

There's a great story floating around the internet from legendary investor Warren Buffett. During a flight, Buffett wanted to lay some wisdom on his personal pilot of ten years, Mike Flint. Trying to help the loyal employee, Buffett asked Flint to craft a list of the twenty-five most important goals he desired in life. After some considerable effort, the pilot thoughtfully created the list.

When Flint presented these goals, Buffet asked him to circle the five which were most important. This put Flint in a deeply introspective state, but after some time he circled the most important goals.

When they sat together to review the list, Buffett asked what Flint's plan was to accomplish these top five goals. The pilot discussed his thoughts and Buffett listened intently.

Then, Buffett asked about the remainder of the pilot's goals.

"Well, the top five are my primary focus, but the other twenty come in at a close second. They are still important so I'll work on those intermittently as I see fit. They are not as urgent, but I still plan to give them a dedicated effort," said the pilot.

Buffett looked the man in the eyes and said,"No. You've got it wrong, Mike. Everything you didn't circle just became your Avoid-At-All-Cost-list. No matter what, these things get no attention from you until you've succeeded with your top five." [2]

Think about how thinly we spread ourselves. If we don't focus on a limited number of incredibly important things, we'll never get a chance to see the finish line. It's ok to have an extended bucket list, but you should have no more than five active goals hovering over your head at any time. Perhaps less.

That level of focus is exactly what brought me to one of the most incredible long-term goals of my own life, and I remember that feeling of finally realizing I had arrived.

Long ago, as a kid, I had an unclear idea of what I wanted to look like. I remember wanting to look heroic like the guys in my favorite movies.

I finally broke it down into an achievable goal using the above blueprint. I wanted to be 9% body fat in less than a year. While the time frame took longer than I had expected (years longer), getting there really blew my mind. As I got closer, it became the only goal on my radar. The rest is history.

Time to write down some goals. Let's get the basics in your transformation journal, and the details can come later as they're needed. Here are the minimum goals I want you to create. Remember, limit your goals to just a few.

- Your long-term weight or body fat % goal.
- The short-term goals that break down your long-term one.
- A challenging fitness goal.
- A book you plan to read related to a personal hero, diet, or fitness (other than this one!).

What is a healthy weight to shoot for? This is different for everybody! You could simply start with the "healthy range" as denoted by the Centers for Disease Control and Prevention (CDC), which can be calculated by Googling "CDC BMI calculator". The algorithm doesn't take into account your unique body characteristics, so don't get too wrapped up in the results. However, the "healthy range" can suffice as a decent enough goal if you don't already have one.

When you create a goal, make sure it's displayed in a prominent place so you can see it and be reminded of it every day. Personally, I have a whiteboard in my bedroom that I see every day. Use whatever works for you. Just remember that life gets busy sometimes, and constant reminders of the things you want to accomplish are a necessity so that you don't get caught up in the day-to-day.

One to two pounds of weight loss per week is an excellent goal, more than that might be trouble, though. Maintaining losses of three or more pounds per week can be really challenging in the long run because it would require a highly restrictive diet. Your motivation will inspire you to bring out the big guns and kick as much butt as you can early on, but your body's rejection mechanism will switch into full gear and will probably bring your progress to a halt before you've made decent headway.

Keep Your Goals to Yourself

Another helpful tip in pursuing your goals is to keep them to yourself. Derek Sivers, entrepreneur and psychology junkie, has spent significant time researching goal setting. In his TED Talk, he suggests that you keep your goals to yourself because the mere act of telling others about your goal gives you a feeling of satisfaction similar to actually obtaining that goal, sapping the drive to complete it.[3]

I looked into the research behind his speech and found a few interesting studies. In summary, they say that we basically obtain satisfaction for our deeds in a few ways. One is a personal belief in accomplishment brought about by making objective gains towards a goal. Another is receiving peer recognition for an accomplishment (apparently regardless of whether it has been achieved).[4] This is contrary to the popular belief that we should announce our intentions to the world so that we're held accountable for our plans.

If, however, you desire to share your goals, Sivers offers a simple way to circumvent the "reward mechanism." Share the work you plan to do to achieve the goal rather than revealing the overarching goal itself. So, instead of "I'm finally going to lose weight this year!" try, "in order to work towards my goal weight, I plan to totally reconfigure my diet and go to the gym three times a week."

FORMING YOUR TRANSFORMATION PLAN

Now that you've got a few goals, how are you going to accomplish them? Your goals are the lighthouse for your plan, guiding the way, but you still need to navigate the rough waters around it.

A transformation plan constitutes the steps that you will take in order to move towards your goals. It will change often, but for now your plan should cover diet and fitness goals. It's easiest to address diet and fitness simultaneously, since effective transformations require both. They are the water and the sunlight that work together to make you grow (or in this case, shrink). For this section of your plan, you will create answers to these questions:

- What is your diet action plan to work towards your goal weight (or bodyfat %)?
- What is your fitness action plan?

Depending on where you are in your own journey, these blueprints will look different. Examples might look like this:

Diet plan

- I will stop drinking soda.
- I will not eat after 6 p.m..

Short-term weight goal

- I will lose one pound by the end of the week.

Long-term weight goal

- I will weigh 200 pounds by December 31st.

Fitness plan

- I will do ten push-ups every morning.
- I will walk around my block (0.5 miles) three days a week.

Diet plan

- I will eat 2,200 calories Monday through Friday.
- I will eat a minimum of 130 grams of protein Monday through Friday.
- I will eat fewer than 200 grams of carbohydrates Monday through Friday.

Short-term weight goal

- I will lose 0.5 pounds by the end of the week.

Long-term weight goal

- I will weigh 170 pounds by December 31st.

Long-term physique goal

- I will be under 12% body fat by December 31st.

Fitness plan

- I will run two miles three times a week.
- I will do strength training, following the ____ plan, four times a week.

"A good plan today is better than a perfect plan tomorrow."

CONRAD BREAN, "WAG THE DOG"

At this point, you have more than enough information to hit the ground running, so create a transformation plan now. If you don't have goals, your plan has holes. Here's the blueprint:

YOUR TRANSFORMATION PLAN

Diet plan
- The thing I plan on doing to lose weight.

Short-term weight goal
- How much weight I want to lose by next week or month.

Long-term weight goal
- How much weight I want to lose by the end of the year, or beyond.

Fitness plan
- The thing I will do to sweat.

With these items completed, there's no need to wait. Start immediately!

My parents and I had a saying, usually as we were about to plow into a plate of junk food: "I'll start my diet tomorrow." We always followed the comment with a chuckle. Screw that!

Take this time to create your own Transformation Plan. It's incredibly important that you create these goals, as well as make some plan for what you intend to do to reach them. Create concrete goals and expect great things of yourself. This is not the time to totally revolutionize your lifestyle and jump in with the big guns blazing. Just take a step, a purposeful expectation of yourself copied your transformation journal. It's a good thing to hold yourself accountable, and perfectly ok for this new responsibility to give you some anxiety. It doesn't have to be daunting, just deliberate.

It's Time for Action

> "Action, action! No other salvation exists. At the beginning was action, also at the end."
>
> —NIKOS KAZANTZAKIS, "ZORBA THE GREEK"

Time to stop being a passive member of your own life. You're not a flesh vessel made to observe the random happenstance of existence, you're here to enjoy what time you have. But time is running out! The only thing that will get you where you want to be is **action.** I'm not talking about the intention of action, I'm talking about literally starting today.

Adopt the mindset of action. Along the way you'll gain knowledge, you'll find better fitness routines, better advice about nutrition, and an all-around better system. However, if you wait for the perfect moment, it will never come.

Here are some thoughts to help inflate the flat tire preventing you from getting the car off the driveway:

- Procrastination will slowly eat away at you.
- Each time you push something off, you **lose** something.
- There are no good excuses.
- You are ready **now**, no matter where you are.
- Time keeps moving. It won't stop and wait for your perfect moment.

The pursuit of a better life and a better self is continuous. Sometimes you'll progress like a raging river, or sometimes like a small babbling brook. After a long enough period of time, even a trickle can transform you.

REPROGRAM YOUR HABITS

"Champions don't do extraordinary things…they do ordinary things, but do them without thinking, too fast for the other team to react. They follow the habits they've learned."

TONY DUNGY QTD. IN "THE POWER OF HABIT: WHY WE DO WHAT WE DO IN LIFE AND BUSINESS" BY CHARLES DUHIGG

Habits are the nuts and bolts of your transformation. When I began my lifestyle transformation, I had lots of negative habits. So many that it was impossible to know where to start.

Throughout the day, nearly every action I made took me further and further away from the man I wanted to become. Each step was a poor choice that compounded into my day-to-day routine. Eventually, to make any headway, I had to rid myself of my negative habits. I replaced them with healthier habits one by one.

Although the habits you have created may hover around in the background, we can create new ones to overcome them. When we build enough of these healthy habits, your course will change towards transformation.

Breaking Down the Habit

I have an aunt that owns a spoon collection. She spent about thirty minutes once (mind you I was twelve) describing what humdrum trip she was on when she found each spoon. Being such a polite kid, I listened quietly, struggling not to openly yawn in front of her.

Later, for some long-forgotten reason, I had to take a seven-hour road trip with her and my uncle. (Who knows what terrible deed I had done for karma to deliver such a blow.)

I couldn't nod off with her high-pitched choir music playing. I could see the beads of sweat on my poor uncle's face as he drove. He probably wanted to open the door and jump out of the moving vehicle just as much as I did.

She had a habit, so I discovered that day, of acquiring a milkshake from every Dairy Queen on the trip that had a sign big enough for her beady little eyes to see. She would inform us of her discovery by proclaiming in an excited manner, "DQ alert, DQ alert!"

Each time my uncle would look at me with desperation, but as a kid, I was fairly excited about my aunt's ice cream addiction, so I joined in on these little pit stops.

On one of them, my uncle decided to partake and ended up spilling half of his milkshake on his shirt. Frustrated with his lot in life, he handed me the rest of it, much to my continued excitement.

My aunt's DQ addiction perfectly describes the mechanics of a habit. I've discovered that the habit loop is arranged in to three simple parts:

cue ➤ routine ➤ reward [1]

The cue was the Dairy Queen sign that she saw as she scanned the horizon. The routine was barking "DQ alert!" to my defeated uncle. Acquiring delicious ice cream followed—to which we enjoyed a sugar-induced chemical high.

I've discovered one benefit to this experience. She has saved me from eating at at least one fast-food chain because every time I see a Dairy Queen, my reaction is to escape the torments of my youth.

What were the specific triggers in her habit loop? Was she looking to get out of the car and stretch? Was she unsatisfied with a lull in the psychological warfare she'd been conducting on my uncle? Were her brain's dopamine receptors relaying their desperation for sugar to her central nervous system? Sometimes it's challenging to identify the components of a habit loop, but a little self-experimentation and perseverance can reveal the things that make us tick.

She had done this enough times that it was an unconscious reaction to seeing the sign. It required no higher-level thought for her because, as I have been told, she'd been doing this for as long as my uncle could remember. This leads us to an important concept.

> "Habits are formed on a conscious level and after enough repetition are reprogrammed to an unconscious part of the brain"

CHARLES DUHIGG, "THE POWER OF HABIT"

Charles Duhigg, the author of *The Power of Habit*, asks: How much concentration did backing out of the driveway take today? Think about learning how to drive, how complex and frustrating it was so long ago. Now you drive home and pay no attention to the actual actions required to operate a vehicle. The habits you have created have been filed into a part of your brain that no longer requires higher-level thought. Luckily so, because you're now free to focus on that bicyclist darting across the street or cleaning up that Dairy Queen milkshake you accidentally dumped on your pants.[1]

A large percentage of the things we do each day are purely habit-based and unconscious. Do you recall if you put your left or right shoe on first, or which limb you dry off first after you get out of the shower? Did you actively think about the route you used to get to work?

Not long ago, I had decided to check out a childhood home, which required a number of turns through a winding and complex neighborhood. I was surprised how easy it was to find it, after having not been there in over ten years.

MIT scientists have found that while we are constantly learning new habits, ones which we've already learned tend to stick around.

"'We've done experiments where we trained rats to run down a maze until it was a habit, and then we extinguished the habit by changing placement of the reward...Then one day, we'll put the reward in the old place, and put in the rat, and, by golly, the old habit will re-emerge right away. Habits never really disappear. They're encoded into the structures of our brain, and that's a huge advantage for us, because it would be awful if we had to relearn how to drive after every vacation. The problem is that your brain can't tell the difference between bad and good habits, and so if you have a bad one, it's always lurking there, waiting for the right cues and rewards.'"

ANN GRAYBIEL,
QTD. IN "THE POWER OF HABIT" BY CHARLES DUHIGG

This can be intimidating, I agree. The bad habits I formed over the years still exist, deep down. Fortunately, they've been replaced by a slew of better ones. Where do you even start? We'll get to it!

Addiction

When my doctor told me as a fat kid that I needed to go on a diet, he didn't really understand my addiction, and for him it was a simple fix. Eat less, move more.

I knew my lifestyle was bad: my heart told me as it skipped beats, my lungs told me as I walked up stairs, my self-respect told me after I saw in the mirror the damage I'd done to myself. I felt like a prisoner, I felt out of control.

What I faced was addiction. The same kind of addiction people suffer from when using drugs and alcohol. Food is tricky, though. You can survive without booze and dope, but you must have food. You have to fuel your body with something!

I recall sitting on the front bench at my dorm in college as a morbidly obese freshman, waiting. For friends, perhaps? No, I was waiting for the pizza delivery guy, and I was hungry! This memory still sticks with me. As I waited, a woman walked up to me and asked if I was all right.

Caught off guard, I responded inquisitively, "yeah, why?"

"Oh, you looked sad is all. I just wanted to see if you were ok," she replied.

I didn't think much of it until later, but the truth about those days is that I *was* sad a lot. I would bring the pizza upstairs to my dark room, watch movies and for a moment feel better. I would feel ok because my body was responding to the chemicals that are released when addicts get their fix.

Studies show that the brain's response to junk food is the same as its response to cocaine and other drugs. [5] When we're exposed to this stimulus over and over, we require increasing amounts to achieve that feeling we have grown to love. Hence my obesity, a runaway train heading full steam towards that broken bridge over the canyon.

I didn't understand the machinery behind my love of food at the time. No wonder I was always having this internal battle. I was at odds because my body had this requirement which, when I attempted to suppress it, responded with its own psychological warfare. I would eventually crawl back to my old ways, giving in to my body's whims only to face more disappointment. What a rough ride it was early on.

Confronting Bad Habits

One of the most challenging hurdles to overcome was the emotional connection I had with food. Studies have shown that heavier people eat excessive amounts of calories compared to normal-weight individuals during times of stress. [6] Often, this is because we rely on food as a coping mechanism. Susan Albers, a psychologist at the Cleveland Clinic and the author of *50 Ways to Soothe Yourself Without Food*, mentions...

> *"Given the strong soothing effect of food on a biological level, we have to work even harder to find ways to soothe and comfort ourselves without calories. This is important in the long run for managing your weight, improving your self-esteem, and protecting your overall health."[7]*

In addition to using food as a coping mechanism, we must also deal with post-binge guilt. Eating binges follow a destructive cycle that looks like this:

stress ➤ comfort-food binge ➤ guilt

How do you break this cycle? In analyzing my own experiences mixed with hours upon hours of research about these topics, the process looks like this:

- Become aware of your habits.
- Break down your habit into cause and effect.
- Consciously decide to change the habit.
- Experiment with changing your routines.
- Practice repetition and positive reinforcement for better habits.

Over years of conditioning, I had allowed an assortment of bad habits to entrench themselves so much in my routine that they created a subconscious machine for their perpetuation. But I failed to give them much consideration. What I did instead was avoid the topic and shrug off the obvious, self-inflicted failure.

Bringing Awareness

> "When I am anxious it is because I am living in the future. When I am depressed it is because I am living in the past."
>
> JIMMY R.

It's so easy to constantly dwell on errors we've made in the past and worry about the things coming tomorrow. With mindfulness, we can chip away at these stresses, but damn it's hard.

The movement towards mindfulness is something I first learned of when reading about Buddhism. A good definition I've found explains mindfulness to be "a state of active, open attention on the present." [8]

A habit is "something that a person does often in a regular and repeated way," usually without thinking. [9] When we can bring awareness to this habit, we are on the path to changing it. Mindfulness is what gives us this awareness. While becoming more mindful, I realized a few of my own bad habits, including:

- Purchasing a massive Big Gulp when I got gas.
- Munching on junk when I watched television.
- Surfing the internet and social media when I was bored.
- Cracking a soda when thirsty. Rarely, if ever, drinking water.
- Incessantly checking my phone and email.
- Buying nachos and a Slurpee at the movie theater.
- Nabbing candy out of the jar at our office secretary's desk throughout the day.

I also noticed I used my emotions to dictate my actions, like unconsciously seeking out some comforting food on my way home from a stressful day of work. I used food as my coping mechanism. But, when I took time to think about my current situation—be it what I ate, how I felt, my exercise routine (or lack thereof), and what actions I did throughout the day—I built awareness.

Rewiring Rewards

Every time you encounter a difficult situation, you can respond in a number of ways. Responding by eating over-processed junk food or mindlessly binging Youtube videos could be holding you back. It's treating a negative symptom with a negative treatment. To fully transform yourself, acquiring healthy coping mechanisms is paramount. It's time to make a mindful decision about the problems you see within yourself. But you must actively decide to change the habit.

Consider these two situations. How will you feel after their conclusions?

Stressful day of work. ➤ Two hours of TMZ, a few items on the dollar menu and a tall glass of Coke.

Stressful day of work. ➤ Walk around the neighborhood, snacking on apple slices with peanut butter while reading a book.

It's easy to think that since you've worked so hard, you deserve the junk food. But that coping mechanism ends up punishing your mind and body. It may feel good at first to indulge, but afterwards, you're faced with guilt and lethargy as you come down from a sugar high. Thinking of these indulgences as rewards creates a cycle that will only reinforce bad habits. You don't need that blow to your health. You deserve better.

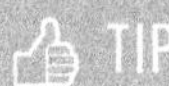 **TIP**

Instead of resorting to eating junk when your days are tough, think of other things that make you happy. Here are a few things that work for me:

- Make a cup of coffee or tea and chill out on a comfy couch.
- Call a friend or family member and have a conversation.
- Go to the gym and exercise for a bit.
- Read something interesting.
- Take a nap.
- Plan a trip or fun activity for the week.
- Watch an episode of your favorite show.
- Blow something up in a video game.
- Go outside and walk around the neighborhood.

Think of items for your own list and **Write It Down**. When you start feeling like heading over to your go-to fast-food joint, you can try an item from the list instead.

Build Keystone Habits

Research suggests that some actions people take can bleed into other areas of transformation. Charles Duhigg, author of *The Power of Habit*, refers to these as "keystone habits." Adopting these few habits might be all you need to rewire your whole way of thinking.

One such keystone habit is writing in a food journal. This important tool allows for keen self-analysis of the habits we may or may not realize we have.

In a research study conducted to observe the effects of food-tracking, scientists discovered that when people were tasked with completing a daily food log, they began to develop heightened awareness.

It wasn't long before some saw patterns in their dieting, and transferred this realization to an actionable habit, like keeping a healthy snack around for mid-morning cravings. It's interesting to note that even though the study had asked the participants to write what they ate only one day a week, people soon used food logging daily as not only a way to keep themselves accountable, but to create a blueprint for un-logged days.

> "...this keystone habit—food journaling—created a structure that helped other habits to flourish. Six months into the study, people who kept daily food records had lost twice as much weight as everyone else."
>
> CHARLES DUHIGG, "THE POWER OF HABIT"

One of the participants mentioned that "after a while, the journal got inside my head. I started thinking about meals differently. It gave me a system for thinking about food without becoming depressed."[1]

But food logging isn't the only key to weight loss. Other habits which are echoed among successful dieters, include:

- Joining a weight loss community.
- Frequent weigh-ins (daily).
- Exercising daily, in the morning if possible.
- Eating a healthy breakfast (if it's part of your plan).
- Having consistent eating patterns. [10]

When asked what his most important habit is for staying healthy and productive, Virgin Mobile CEO Richard Branson says exercise. He goes on to say, "I definitely can achieve twice as much in a day by keeping fit."[11]

What keystone habits will make it all click for you? Everybody is different, so experiment with some ideas and be open to new ones.

👍 TIP

An essential keystone habit I found was a deep curiosity for health and fitness. This caused my knowledge to bloom exponentially, and I can thank all of the information on the internet, YouTube, and in books and magazines for that. Being a lifelong learner has upgraded my efforts for a healthy life repeatedly.

Likewise, if you never stop learning, you'll find the keystone habit of continuous self-education to be as vital as I have.

Create a Re-action Plan

> "Once you understand that habits can be rebuilt, the power of habit becomes easier to grasp, and the only option left is to get to work."
>
> CHARLES DUHIGG, "THE POWER OF HABIT"

Once you decide to become aware of your habits and find a few you want to change, you might find it helpful to create a re-action plan.

Decide how you are going to replace the negative response with a positive one. This is highly individual, and I encourage you to customize it to your needs. I'll provide a blueprint with a few examples.

To understand the habit better, spend a week trying to learn about it before you really work on changing it. First, identify the cue, or the thing that triggers the habit. In the story about my aunt, her cue was seeing the Dairy Queen sign. That alone set off her feverish ice-cream frenzy.

For you, the things that initiate a bad habit may not be so obvious. Duhigg recommends carrying a journal with you and making note of five things each time you notice an undesirable craving or habit:

- Where are you?
- What time is it?
- How are you feeling?
- Who is around you?
- What are you doing at that moment? [1]

If this process enables you to see a trend, there might be a simple fix.

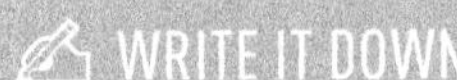

WRITE IT DOWN

When you identify a habit you want to change, create a re-action plan. Grab your transformation journal. On the left hand page you will create the blueprint, and the opposite side is where you'll keep track of your progress.

RE-ACTION PLAN BLUEPRINT

Habit I will change:

What is the cue?

What is my new routine going to be?

If the craving still exists, what else can I do?

RE-ACTION PLAN PROGRESS

Habit I will change: Staying up really late watching Netflix.

What is the cue? Before bed, I always turn on the television to watch something while I'm brushing my teeth and getting ready to sleep.

What is my new routine going to be? Instead of turning on the television right before bed, I'll just watch an hour of it after I get home from work if I want to catch up on something. The period of time when I am preparing to sleep will be a no-TV time.

If the craving still exists, what else can I do? I will read a book while lying in bed.

Habit I will change: Grabbing a McDonald's Frappe on my way home from work.

What is the cue? Getting in my car, I notice a strong urge to drive to the McDonald's on the way home and grab my blended coffee treat.

What is my new routine going to be? I will make a cup of tea to sip on before I get in my car.

If the craving still exists, what else can I do? I will eat a handful of almonds before I get in my car and head home, possibly using a different route.

On the right hand page (or near the re-action plan), keep track of your progress by writing an **X** for successful re-actions. If you mess up you don't have to write anything down (the guilt of seeing a bad mark will be a bummer to see). Use this technique for however long you need. Awareness combined with a constructive alternate plan will provide a good system for changing your habits.

Make a re-action plan for habits you want to change, but start small. Do your best to hold yourself accountable for the decisions you make, because this only works if you put in the effort.

> "It seems ridiculously simple, but once you're aware of how your habit works, once you recognize the cues and rewards, you're halfway to changing it."
>
> NATHAN AZRIN,
> QTD. IN "THE POWER OF HABIT" BY CHARLES DUHIGG

Forming New Habits

After all we've learned so far, forming new habits is easy as pie. Remember the mechanics of a habit: there is the cue or trigger, the action itself, and the reward you obtain from it.

If you attempt to form a new, and better, habit with this system, you'll make it easier on yourself because you're designing it so that your brain will be trained to execute it unconsciously. Pushing it to an unconscious part of the brain is good too because it gives you less opportunity to think about the reasons why you shouldn't be doing it in the first place!

Let's say you want to start a new exercise habit in the morning. Let's design a cue, routine, and reward.

Cue: Waking up and seeing laid-out workout clothes, drinking a cup of water, listening to some high energy tunes.

Routine: Tearing up the streets with your morning run.

Reward: Endorphins, positive vibes, self-confidence. A big cup of your favorite coffee, and homemade breakfast.

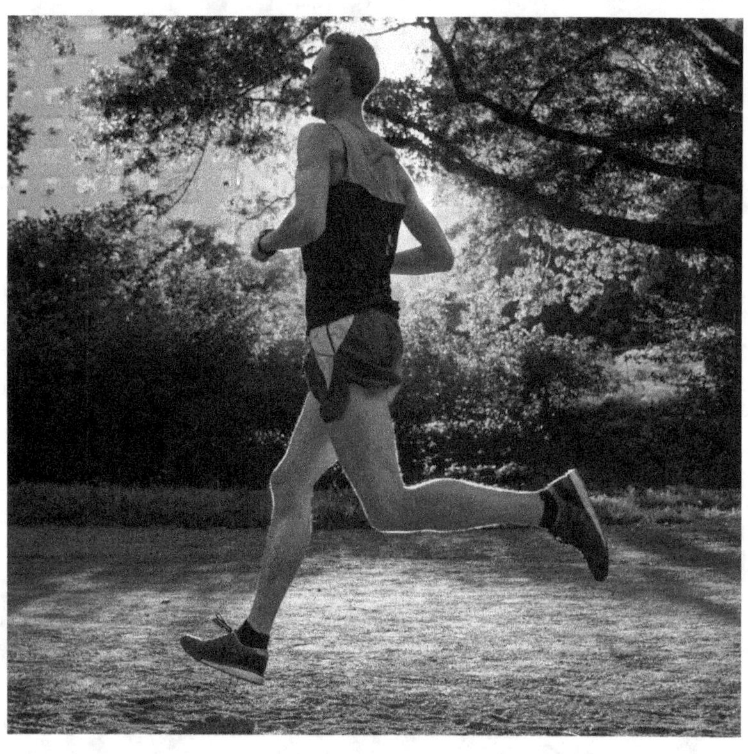

Eventually, you'll connect your morning routine with exercise. The more senses you involve, the more impactful the cue will be.

> "Treat The Gym Like A Spa. Yes. It has to feel good. I tell people this a lot, go to the gym, and just sit there, and read a magazine, and then go home. And do this every day. Go to the gym, don't even work out. Just GO. Because the habit of going to the gym is more important than the workout. [...] There are times when, I'm not even kidding, there are times when I'm in the middle of a workout, and actually woke up because I am so ingrained with going to the gym and being there, it's that much of a habit to me. The first thing I do in the morning is work out. I lay out my workout clothes the night before, and just hop in 'em. So lay out your clothes, and go to the gym, and relax. HAHAHAHA! But sooner or later, you WILL work out."
>
> *TERRY CREWS, IN AN AMA (ASK ME ANYTHING) ON REDDIT.COM*

The X Effect

I've found an effective way to promote habit formation called the X Effect. Introduced by a member of the Reddit community in 2014, it gained a large following shortly thereafter and is undoubtedly one of the best outlines I've seen for acquiring new habits, one I've used myself to great success.[12]

Here's the premise: You dream up the habit you want to form, hold yourself accountable day-to-day with a calendar and red pen to mark successful completions, and continue this for a couple of months. I've taken the technique and simplified it, here are the steps:

1. Purchase or print out a monthly calendar.

2. Think of a new habit you want to form (start small) and write it on the start date.

3. Start immediately. When you have successfully completed the habit for the day, mark a large X on the box associated with that day (ideally with a red pen) and continue marking an X daily until you have fully completed two months. By the end, you will likely have built the habit into your subconscious.

4. If you miss a day, you MUST complete the task the next day. Also, don't write in the X for the day you missed.

5. If you miss two days, make a smaller goal and start over.

6. Each habit should have its own calendar, and it works best when you can see the whole month on one page.

One study suggests that the time it takes to form a new habit is somewhere around sixty-six days, but this varies from person to person and habit to habit.[13] Doing things this way will definitely propel you to a more solid foundation for the habit.

Since the conception of this idea, habit tracking has become mainstream. You might find that an existing cell phone habit tracking app can better fit your lifestyle, especially if you desire to go paperless.

Instinct

What is the end result of so effortfully deconstructing and replacing your habits? One word: instinct. When a habit becomes instinct, it has graduated to the next level. It's when you create instincts that things really feel easier. You're not always going to need to live by a blueprint because, eventually, making the right choices will happen naturally, unconsciously. What seems so difficult now, won't always be so.

FORGING A NEW RELATIONSHIP WITH FOOD

When I was ten years old, my family moved to Reno, Nevada, the biggest little city in the world.

Things weren't easy for my parents during this time, jobs apparently weren't so plentiful for my pops, and my mom ended up having to take a job out in California and fly back and forth when she could. It was unsustainable. For the short-time we were there (a little over a year and a half) we were in survival mode.

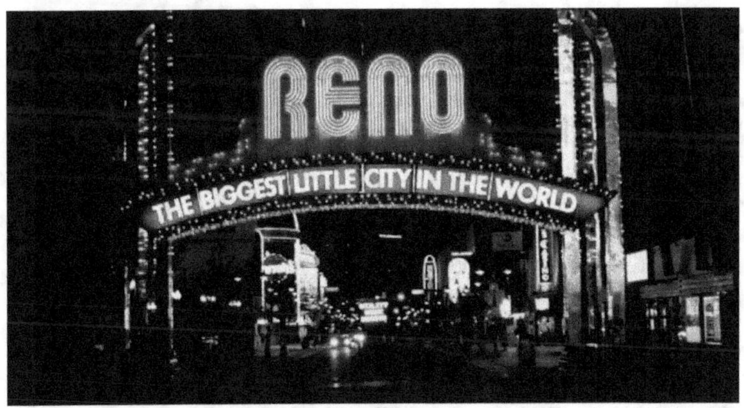

When we *were* together, it was blowout time. When we would go out, we hit the casinos, where one small family could eat to their heart's content for less than twenty bucks.

Fullness felt safe; it felt like we were ok. Fullness creates such an instinctually calming feeling. Our bodies don't understand the concerns of the modern world, but when the belly is full, something deep inside us gives assurances.

Fullness became the thing that let me know things were alright. With my parents on the verge of divorce, my kid world was seemingly stitched together by a rapidly weakening thread. But in those moments of peace at the dinner table, we could be together basking in the euphoria of a full tummy, feeling remarkably happy. And so, happiness and food became intertwined; food made me happy and fullness made me feel safe. Who wouldn't want to feel happy and safe all the time?

Fullness became some sort of psychological trigger, and the harder it was pressed, the better things felt. It was almost competitive at times; our family only put away three platters of ribs at the Mining Camp restaurant? Not bad, but we can do better. If I didn't have cramps in my sides, and could speak in complete sentences, I had wasted my time at the Circus Circus Casino buffet.

Reprogramming the Relationship

Oftentimes, it's intimidating to have to consider giving up the thing that keeps you safe and happy. For a lot of us who struggle with weight, this thing is food. You might think you'd have to give it all up and move to an isolated island colony to eat seaweed and clams for the rest of your life, free from temptation, but it's definitely possible to take care of business right at home.

In this section, we're going to sweep out some old ideas, not under the rug, but out the door. This is a foundational section. You're not going to find all the information you might want in your grand quest, that's not my goal, but in this day and age it's extremely important to freshen up the mindset we have about food. We are force-fed bad info at ridiculous proportions, so it's more important than ever to sift through the slop and create your own path. Food should be our friend.

Breaking the Cycle

Up to this point, we've uncovered a system for breaking the cycle. You'll see this system's relevance in many ways, here we can relate it to the cycle of poor diet choices.

Eating the wrong way was one of the biggest things I did to keep me fat. Once I started to correct the course, everything started to change. Here is a recap of the things we've learned so far:

1. Create goals. Look at them every day.

2. Actually decide to act a certain way and then put in conscious effort.

3. Be realistic with your expectations and take baby steps.

4. Manage cravings by observing the habit and break the cycle with better alternatives.

What does it take to snap out of the cycle of failed diet attempts? The problem partly stems from skipping the basics. If you fail to define what you want to accomplish (in the proper goal format) and fail to make a real plan, you probably won't get as far as you'd like. But stopping there will mean you're missing a ton! In this chapter, I'll reveal more effective techniques that will lead you to success. Firstly, what is real food?

Real Food

Real food is the good stuff that is grown or raised as opposed to processed and engineered. Our bodies are poorly adapted to eat too much of the refined food so widely available today.

Real food is nutrient-rich, natural, and simple. If it was grown from the ground or raised with care, you're on the right path.

What makes real food preferable to processed, prepackaged, or fast-food meals is:

- You know the ingredients.
- It's loaded with vitamins and nutrients.
- It doesn't spike your blood sugar as much (for the most part).
- It's generally lower in calories by volume.
- It's easier to track.
- You have maximum control.

Beyond understanding what real food is, we need to comprehend the mentality behind real food. Moving towards making real food a part of your life is not just about staving off disease or aiding your weight goals, it's about self-reliance. It's about being more mindful of the fuel that runs your body.

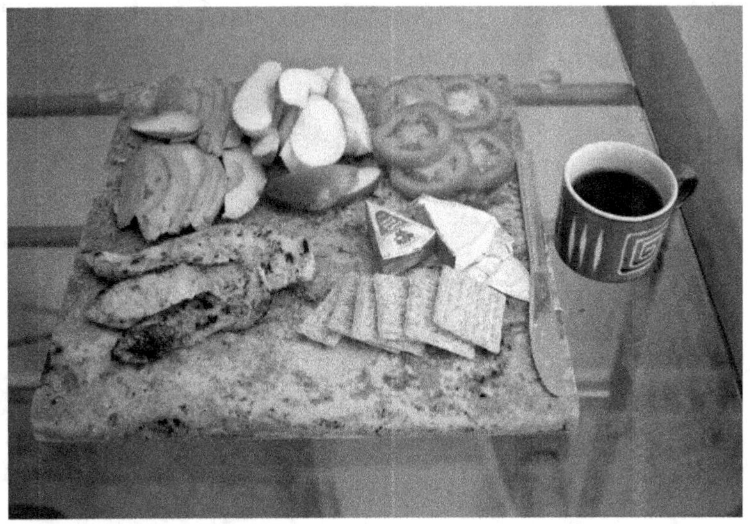

Food Guidelines

"Food is one of life's greatest joys yet we've reached this really sad point where we're turning food into the enemy, and something to be afraid of. I believe that when you use good ingredients to make pasta dishes, salads, stews, burgers, grilled vegetables, fruit salads, and even outrageous cakes, they all have a place in our diets. We just need to rediscover our common sense: if you want to curl up and eat macaroni and cheese every once in a while – that's alright! Just have a sensible portion next to a fresh salad, and don't eat a big old helping of chocolate cake afterwards."

JAMIE OLIVER,
"JAMIE OLIVER'S FOOD REVOLUTION"

I don't know what the one optimal human diet is. Neither do the people with a lot more initials after their name. The more that I learn, the more it seems we're all designed differently. What our bodies are optimally adapted for can significantly depend on our genetic and geographical background.

Studies have shown that colon size can vary in lengths upwards of five feet between people of different regions. [14] Given that the gut is the organ responsible for absorbing food, something about their diets and the associated survival advantage facilitated this change.

Some groups of individuals are also able to tolerate more milk in their diets by having an increased production of lactase, an enzyme that breaks lactose (milk sugars) down before it causes uncomfortable gassy situations.[15] Beyond that, the bacteria in your colon that participate in this breaking down of foods can vary significantly from one region to the next.[16]

The takeaway from all this is that, depending on a host of factors, your body may be predisposed to processing foods in a different way than the fella hanging out next to you at the coffee shop.

Now, you're probably thinking, "Great! thanks for all the TMI, but what are we supposed to do with this?"

Well, it's simple. **We can eat a diverse selection of real food, and follow a few rules that work for the majority of people.** Don't worry, this lifestyle isn't complicated, thank goodness...

Let's start by bulldozing some of the common diet misconceptions. The dieting no-no list below is by no means comprehensive, but a good start nonetheless.

Dieting No-Nos:

- Cleanses and detox plans that aren't indicated by a legit healthcare professional (our body does a pretty good job of detoxing itself).
- Excessive anything.
- Liquid diets.
- The cold turkey tactic. Eliminating treats and sweets completely.
- Eating most of your food on the go.
- Getting a significant amount of your calories from fast-food chains.
- Diets that don't allow for some degree of flexibility.
- Diet systems that take away control (pre-packaged).
- Focusing heavily on supplements.
- Using weight loss pills (a dubious industry at best).
- Diets that aren't supported by science.
- Starving yourself (severe low-calorie dieting).
- Weight loss centers that utilize hormone injections and 500 calorie-per-day diets (they exist!).

At the end of the day, we're looking for a sensible and realistic approach. Losing the chub is one thing, but it is possible to gear yourself up for a lifestyle that promotes things other than weight loss.

Long-term health is the ultimate goal of reprogramming your relationship with food, not just weight loss. Weight loss is just one of the many good side effects of eating right. Dieting is a tool that works so long as it's being used, but who wants to diet for all of eternity? If you adopt healthy eating habits, you won't have to *diet* to maintain your healthy weight once you achieve it.

With short-term "diets," odds are greatly in favor of a weight relapse. Without efforts to obtain fresh eating habits, you'll boomerang back into the same old ways once the diet is finished.

Below are some of the basic improvements that have allowed me to maintain my health and current weight with ease. I like to call them my:

Food Commandments

- Natural ingredients (real food without preservatives, added sugars, or refined materials).
- Diet consisting mostly of plant-based foods.
- Home-cooked meals the majority of the time.
- Meal-prepping for life on the go.
- A wide range of different foods.
- Flexibility that allows for splurges or treats now and then.
- Utilizing healthy snacks when needed.
- Low/no calorie liquids (sparkling water & black coffee are my favorites).

👍 TIP

In a perfect world, all beef would be grass-fed, all salmon would be caught from babbling forest streams, and all chickens would be raised running free in a sunny barnyard. I would love to have my fridge stocked with the best foods at all times, but it doesn't always happen.

Philosophically, I agree with keeping things better, more sustainable, and more natural. But I don't always walk that path, and for the majority of us, what matters is not that everything we eat is organic, free-range, and non-GMO, but that we try to eat foods that are produced better, and support local farming when we can.

Following these simple food commandments, most people will easily shed some excess weight. It's very important to know that you do not need to trick, fool, confuse, or disorient your body to lose weight. I frequently read about intriguing ways to overcomplicate the crap out of the pretty simple act of eating right. Simplicity is key!

Hara Hachi Bu

As I've leveled up in my questline for health, I've found a few new mindsets that provide me quicker access to my goals. Feeling full all the time saps me of energy, and is usually a keen indicator of overeating. Ditch the ball and chain of a stretched stomach; it's time to take on a new philosophy of eating.

Back in the day, fullness was once a competitive game to me. I recall comparing how many plates of food my cousins and I had dominated in a buffet run, where the tallest stack claimed victory. But the more prestigious we were in the eyes of our heavyset club, the sicker we became. Our support system pushed a lifestyle that was bringing us, one stack of plates at a time, to a ruinous end.

My support system had it wrong, but there are some folks that eat more sensibly. In the southernmost prefecture of Japan, a large concentration of centenarians thrive to this day. A centenarian is an individual who has reached 100 years of age and one of the populations with the highest ratio of these centenarians is in Okinawa. A team of scientists has been collecting data on this population for over twenty years now. These studies are aimed at trying to understand what cultural habits lead to this longevity. Of the unique behaviors they observed was something called "hara hachi bu," which is roughly translated as "eat until eight-parts full" (out of ten).[17]

This is one of the ways the Okinawans have been able to keep their eating in check and fight the natural human instinct to pig out in abundance. Since we're such a modern society, we're almost always in abundance. The feast and famine instinct just doesn't serve us as it once did.

How do we even know where eight out of ten is? It can be discovered through a practice called mindful eating. Mindfulness can be supported with a few tips that help us remove distractions and turn up the volume on what our body is trying to tell us.

Eating Mindfully:

- Eat in a quiet setting, turning off the television.
- Use portion control devices (like smaller plates, and specifically sized containers for meals on the go). Your eyes are always bigger than your stomach, as the idiom goes.
- Slow down the shoveling, and put down your utensil after each bite. Eating slowly lets the *feeling* of fullness come before we've ravenously plowed through extra servings.
- Cook with love, and learn to appreciate the flavors of the things you make.
- Sit down to a table after all the items are prepared, as opposed to grazing in the kitchen while parts of the meal are cooking.

The goal is the feeling of being pleasantly full, not regretfully stuffed. Or, to think of it in another way: we need to wait for our body to signal to us we're full, hormonally, and not try to feel full, physically.

> 👍 TIP
>
> Some foods have a more satiating effect. I could eat an entire dump truck of caramel popcorn and still feel hungry, but if I have a scoop or two of peanut butter, I'm good to go. Dr. Jason Fung of *The Obesity Code* states that "there are natural satiety hormones (peptide YY, cholecystokinin) that respond to protein and fat. Eating pure carbohydrate does not activate these systems and leads to overconsumption."[18]

Home-Cooked Meals and Meal Prep

Kai Greene, IFBB pro bodybuilder, and multiple time Mr. Olympia frontrunner states that "a critical tool for getting ahead in this game of preparation is Tupperware."[19] It doesn't matter whether you're training for a bodybuilding competition or just transforming yourself to be leaner and healthier. Meal preparation makes life easier.

The habit of being more methodical about what we eat can help us get locked into our plan. For the busiest of us, this is not only beneficial but downright required for reaching our goals.

One of the super cool things that patients like to do at the hospital where I work is to thank the staff by bringing treats. These treats are things like cookies, doughnuts, candy, and pastries. If that wasn't enough, we always seem to be throwing a potluck for someone's birthday, or some holiday. Any chance to splurge, we usually take it!

Perhaps the breakroom at your place of employment has a similar situation. I know mine can get out of control. With the accessibility of all these tasty treats, I make sure I have a plan the second I step into the unit. While I'm not always perfect in my adherence to this plan, meal prepping makes a huge difference.

I also like to exercise another percentage rule, the 90/10 rule in dieting. This rule states that when I am on target 90% of the time, I can eat what I want the other 10%. [20] I spin it like this, because if I eat like a pro during my work week, I can splurge now and then on the weekend. Meal prepping has become the way to obtain this level of flexibility. I'll outline my simple system.

When do you meal prep? Personally, I like to do it at the end of my series of days off, or for the Monday-to-Friday crowd, this would be Sunday. You could just do it each night before your workday, but my job is exhausting and I typically don't have a lot of inspiration after a busy day. Break out your Tupperware containers and line them all up for each workday, then start cooking!

If you only stick to the typical grilled chicken or tilapia with broccoli arrangement you'll start believing you're in a prison of your own making with flavorless particle board walls. I suggest going above and beyond this utilitarian plate. If the meals are appetizing, you will be much less likely to be tempted by Karen's going-away potluck. As an added benefit, you'll learn to cook (if you haven't already)! A quick google search for "meal prep ideas" will give you a lifetime's worth of things to try.

So, what exactly do I meal prep for? Anything and everything. This could be your food for the entire day, or just the food you'll eat at work. It doesn't even have to be for anything specific at all; having a few frozen "emergency" meals around is always a good idea.

Most of my meal prepping is for work, and I cook my other meals at home where it has become an integral part of the warm-up and cool-down phases of my days. I find the act of cooking to be soothing and enjoy the habit of spending time with some good tunes playing or having a few laughs with my family. These behaviors help associate positive vibes with the process.

Eating your calories with fibrous foods slows down food absorption. This is partially why fruit, being carb-rich, is usually ok for eating while trying to lose weight.[21]

I break meals down into three components. Protein, starch, and veggies. I generally like to portion my plates in this fashion for simplicity sake, nothing precise or complicated about it.

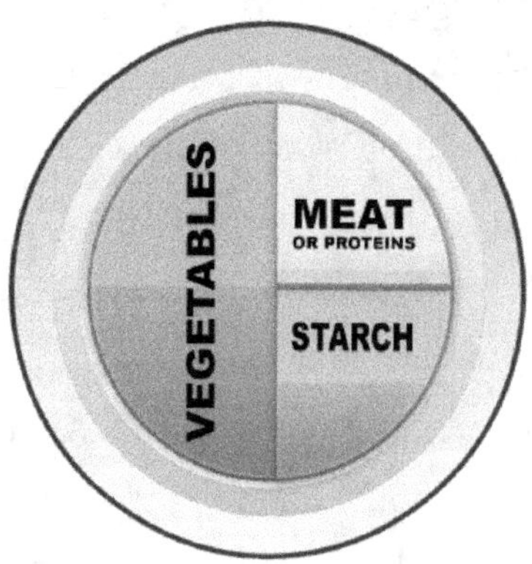

The Meal Prep Pipeline

Let's take a peek at the production line for my typical meal prepping. I like to keep things organized per day, and line the Tupperwares up similarly.

The containers I use are four-cup (thirty-two ounce), single compartment versions. I personally like this size because it gets me to that 8/10 spot that we're shooting for.

Weigh out all your portions (if calorie counting) and drop them in systematically. (Store all your items in a grocery bag or your lunch box the night before.)

A typical shopping run should consist of varied items that help make the meals more interesting and include a wide variety of basic whole foods. Sometimes it's just fun to grab something you've never used before and deal with the how-to of cooking it after bringing it home. (I still haven't figured out how the hell to make eggplant tasty.)

After some sorting, and cooking, the end result of the production line has all my foods lined up ready for individual day packaging.

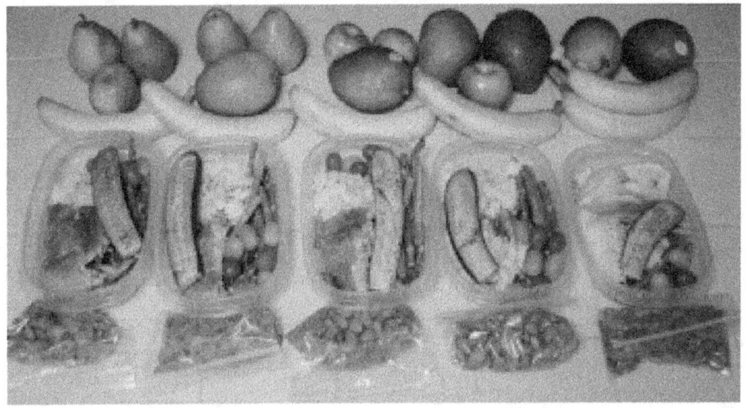

Snacks to the Rescue

Snacks are a great tool. If used effectively, they can help you keep your wits about you throughout the day. I choose snacks that are easy on my blood sugar, healthy, and transportable.

With a good stock of items at home, I'm able to have a snack plan for wherever my day takes me. You're not likely to find me without a baggie of almonds or an apple, even if I'm only headed to the coffee shop for a few hours. I've broken down my snack system into three categories: grazing, break, and breakthrough snacks.

Grazing snacks: For me, this consists of a bag of nuts, almonds, walnuts, macadamia nuts, or maybe even soy nuts or freeze-dried chickpeas.

Having something to peck at throughout the day to instill little nuggets of nutrition helps keep your mind sharp on the tasks at hand without having to worry about your tummy barking too much.

Break snacks: I want to talk about a little thing I call the apple break. I think it's one of the most magical moments in my workday. It consists of two parts: gingerly eating an apple, and not thinking about much. It's like apple-meditation. This is a healthier equivalent to a smoke break, and I really rely on them to help keep my mind in a zen-like state after a mad rush of business, or any time I think I need it.

You can use any transportable snack. Most fruit does well to fit this category. But I like my apples, and always bring a few to work. If you give yourself a super-small mental vacation, and do it while reinforcing healthy eating habits, you'll start to believe in the power of the apple break.

Breakthrough snacks: The breakthrough snack is a tightly packaged little nugget of nutrition designed to be cracked into when you've exhausted your other snacks, and even after you've had your meal. It keeps your head cool when your stomach starts to convince you that the break room full of junk food is worth giving a once over.

Its importance is that it has a mix of calories that put out the initial hunger fire and are also going to give you sustained satiety. I like to think of this as a 'baby' meal in a sense, and it usually consists of a protein shake for me (although there are other options).

Here's a cool thing about your standard protein powder, it comes in two general setups: casein, and whey. These are the byproducts of cheese production and are full-spectrum proteins that cover all the bases we need. Our body absorbs whey protein pretty quickly, and absorbs casein protein a bit slower because it 'gels' up in the stomach after ingestion. [22] A fairly common practice for bodybuilders is to drink casein protein at night before bed so that they are not without nutrition during their typically fasted sleep state. This ideology can be utilized for snacking too!

Whatever you use, make sure it's going to take a while to digest so that you can keep your eyes on the prize all the way home in time for dinner.

- There are vegan protein powder options for those who are inclined to eat such diets, which usually include proteins derived from soy, peas, brown rice, or occasionally from nuts and seeds (like sunflower, hemp, or chia).
- Check out powdered peanut butter (oil content removed) for a protein/flavor boost in a smoothie. Or plain old peanut butter is also pretty excellent. (Sunflower butter is a good alternative for those with nut allergies).

- Soylent is a very interesting meal replacement drink with a full range of nutrients, vitamins, and minerals. There are people actually living off of this stuff, which I wouldn't endorse, but individually packaged drinks have four hundred calories. It's not a bad way to snack on the go; formulations of it now even contain coffee for that caffeine boost.

As a disclaimer, there are some experts that suggest we eliminate snacking altogether. Constantly stimulating our body with calories causes an elevation in fat storage hormones (insulin) and can potentially hinder our progress. While I utilized healthy snacks often in my own transformation, your experience might be different.

Let's review, shall we? We've learned the benefits of real food, and understand that our tummies need not be brought to pant-stretching limits. We will know our limits because we are going to be more mindful of our eating during our meal times, and listen to our bodies.

Since we meal prep, we can eat on the go, and never be without quality meals. This is an awesome place to be, because you are now on the right track! Eventually though, you'll need to add a few more weapons to the arsenal to fight a new foe, the weight loss plateau.

Rest easy friend, plateaus happen to us all at different stages in our adventure.

Here's how we end their reign of terror.

Dealing with the Plateau

The plateau is a stagnation in weight loss. Plateaus were a common occurrence for me. Sometimes I just linked my blow-it days too closely together, but sometimes I did everything right and the scale didn't budge. Your body sure can try to maintain weight, but these mechanisms can be defeated.

In this section, we will go over the process for troubleshooting your diet in a general sense, as well as providing some tips and techniques to get you out of the lull.

When I experience a weight loss plateau, I use a six-phase process that helps build control and awareness.

Phase 1: Build Awareness

The first phase in defeating a plateau is to build awareness. I like what Terry Crews has to say on the topic.

> "For 30 days, I won't 'diet,' but I write down everything I eat, no matter how small. Usually, if I know it's bad and know I have to write it down, I won't eat it."
>
> *TERRY CREWS*

There was a study that tested this technique during one of the most difficult dieting times of the season: Christmas to New Years. Individuals were enrolled in a weight loss program, in which half of the participants were told to 'self-monitor' by completing diet journals and the other half were not.

The individuals who self-reported lost an average of two pounds during this timeframe, and the rest gained an average of two pounds.[23] Other such studies have also confirmed how important and powerful self-monitoring can be.

Below is the template I personally use for building awareness, it's very important to include drinks that have calories in them as well as your exercise for the day. I'm not suggesting writing down calories, just to keep a log of calorie containing foods and drinks.

	MON	TUE	WED	THU
WEIGHT				
MEAL 1				
MEAL 2				
MEAL 3				
SNACKS				
EXERCISE				

Tracking your meals and workouts helps you understand your day-to-day food and fitness habits. Awareness will help you make better choices if you realize you have to **Write It Down,** like Terry Crews suggests!

If you're not ready to keep track of everything you're eating, you should at least use this technique during high-risk periods including holidays, vacations, or other food-filled events or seasons.

On top of tracking your foods, track your body with the three-point measurement system. While the scale is the standard for which we base our weight loss goals, it is inaccurate for day-to-day changes, especially if we're eating a meal high in sodium (sudden water weight increases are a bummer). This is why it's important to measure your progress with these extra steps.

Inaccurate as it can be, I do recommend a daily check-in with your weight (unless the inevitable fluctuations give you anxiety). Conversely, visual and tape measurement changes will happen so slowly that you won't need to do those more than monthly. Easier yet might be to measure and photograph yourself at five to ten pound increments on your weight loss journey.

Three-point transformation measurement system:
- Weight via bathroom scale.
- Tape measurements of specific spots.
- Photographs of yourself in various poses.

You can obtain a cloth tape measure from any large grocery store or Amazon.com, and use it to keep track of various key points in your body. The most important measurement is your waist and hips, as they're usually the places where changes are most obvious and less prone to human error while measuring (the belly button is a good measurement point). I recommend measuring other spots too.

Here are some common spots that I used.

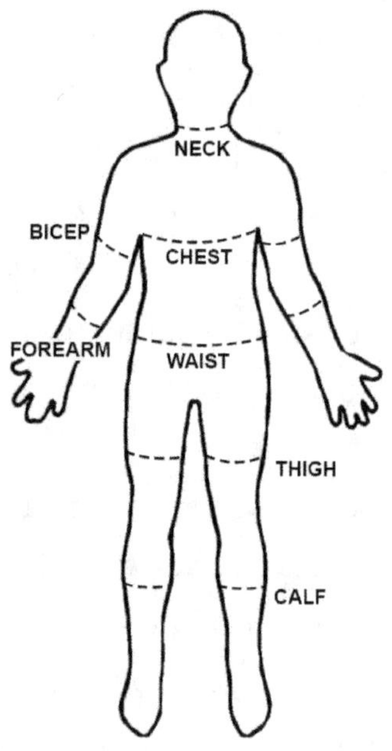

Next, take photographs! They will be your transformation resume, and looking back will be one of the most shocking identifiers of how far you've come. I am so very glad I spent the time taking photographs and oftentimes look at them just to reminisce.

At a minimum, take pictures standing facing forward with your arms down, as well as a side profile. I recommend you take all sorts of poses, the more the merrier. For each update, take the pictures from the same spot, and stand at the same distance. Photographs from different heights and distances can give you a false sense of proportion.

Phase 2: Are Your Blow-it Meals Killing Progress?

Early on, it's acceptable and sometimes even recommended to allow for more leeway with your diet. This involves blow-it meals, blow-it days, or other such treats that don't really fit into the diet program but are allowed to help with your sanity. I utilized blow-it meals in one form or another for a lot of my transformation, although sometimes they can be temporary progress killers.

Blow-it meals will create a saw tooth pattern in your weight loss, as demonstrated in the graphs below.

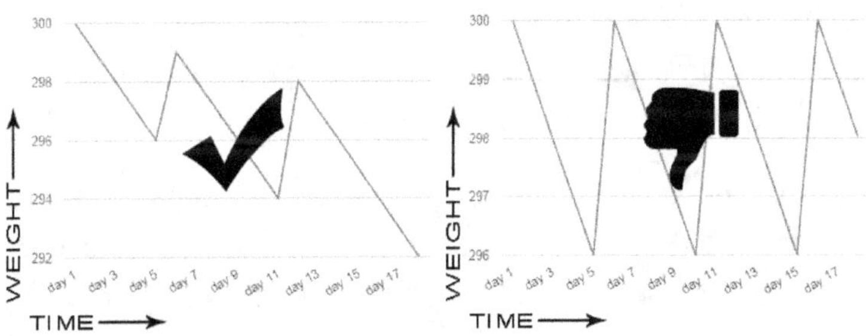

Make sure that the blow-it days aren't crippling your journey and bringing you back, week to week, to the same Monday starting weight.

👍 TIP

If you have a blow-it day, try to take it outside your home. If you do eat at home, make sure it's all gone by the next day so you don't have any pressure to extend the pig-out. I'm not suggesting you bust a seam trying to fit it all in, you can donate leftovers to the break room at work, a friend, or a homeless fella.

Phase 3: Cutting Carbs

Sooner or later you're going to hear about the evils of carbohydrates. True, not all carbs are bad, but bad carbs are really bad. So much so that they're the fattest punching bag for the latest generation of diet advice.

> "...the precise foods responsible for making us fat are also the ones we're likely to rank highest on a list of foods we crave and would never want to live without—pasta, bagels, bread, French fries, sweets, and beer among them.
>
> This is not a coincidence. It's clear from animal research that the foods animals will preferentially eat perhaps to excess are those that most quickly supply energy to the cells—easily digestible carbohydrates."
>
> GARY TAUBES, "WHY WE GET FAT"

Nutritional science has been through 100-plus years of troubleshooting, and what we've learned is that a diet with an excess of fast-digesting carbs will seriously handicap your ability to shed fat. This is mostly why diets that significantly reduce carbs work so well, such as Atkins/Keto (very low carb), and Paleo style (eating like a caveman).

If you want to really supercharge your weight loss, cut out the common bad-carb vices a lot of us have. They include:

- Soda and fruit juice.
- Candy.
- Dessert.
- Chips and snack-y junk food.
- Processed fast-food.
- Decadent coffee drinks (Frappuchinos).
- Bread, tortillas, and other flour-based stuff.

Picking away at the food vices we have is a great way to move away from our psychological, addictive nature towards things that our body doesn't need anyways. Replacing our old food vices with newer, healthy ones is the way to go. Here are some of the things I've adopted:

- Soda can be replaced with coffee or tea.
- Dessert can be replaced with fruit.
- Chips can be replaced with nuts, popcorn, or fruit.
- Candy can be replaced with sugar-free gum.

Come up with your own healthy options to the food vices you have so that you can whittle them out as you progress with your transformation.

👍 TIP

Drink your coffee and tea without sugar or milk. This is an excellent exercise in restraint, and if you're a coffee or tea drinker, one you need to test yourself with. If you disassociate your sippy drinks with the sweetness they're so often accompanied with, you will have an excellent distraction for when you *do* get cravings. I get similar satisfaction from drinking a good cup of black coffee that I get when I eat something delicious, and that really helps in situations where my willpower might otherwise bend.

Phase 4: Step Up Your Fitness Game

Cutting out certain food vices and tightening up your self-monitoring will likely get you back on the wagon to weight loss. Resorting to stricter practices shouldn't be utilized early on, so save calorie counting as a last resort (unless your brain is really wired for it).

Likewise, when you're getting started, burning 100 calories on the treadmill can seem daunting. But as you improve your fitness capabilities, you'll find that sweating out that amount of calories becomes easier and easier. Eventually, you'll be able to really get into a groove, and the calorie burn that you achieve can be bigger and longer-lasting.

As an extreme example, Olympic medalist Michael Phelps has been reported to have a 12,000 calorie diet during his training days (the typical person eats between 2,000-3,000 calories a day). Here's an account of a typical day in the life of his stomach.

> "Phelps lends a new spin to the phrase "Breakfast of Champions" by starting off his day by eating three fried-egg sandwiches loaded with cheese, lettuce, tomatoes, fried onions and mayonnaise.
>
> He follows that up with two cups of coffee, a five-egg omelet, a bowl of grits, three slices of French toast topped with powdered sugar and three chocolate-chip pancakes.
>
> At lunch, Phelps gobbles up a pound of enriched pasta and two large ham and cheese sandwiches slathered with mayo on white bread – capping off the meal by chugging about 1,000 calories worth of energy drinks.
>
> For dinner, Phelps really loads up on the carbs – what he needs to give him plenty of energy for his five-hours-a-day, six-days-a-week regimen – with a pound of pasta and an entire pizza.
>
> He washes all that down with another 1,000 calories worth of energy drinks."

NEW YORK TIMES [24]

As I'm sure you've seen, his physique is impressive and lean. It's through his incredible calorie-burning swimming sessions (and equally amazing genetics) that he prevents himself from looking like a manatee instead.

Now, I'm not suggesting you make your life about sleeping, eating, and working out (and probably pooping a lot).

But running an extra few miles, and doing a few more sets at the gym will definitely add up over the long run, and might nudge you through a plateau. As your strength and endurance increases, it's natural to want to do more and try new things.

> "Humans evolved as a species that walks, runs, climbs trees and hills, and uses a variety of muscles all the time. Now people use elevators and escalators instead of stairs, drive instead of walk, use dishwashers and washing machines instead of washing dishes and clothes by hand, buy food instead of growing it, and hire people to do even minor repair work around the house instead of fixing things ourselves."
>
> DR. VALTER LONGO, "THE LONGEVITY DIET"

👍 TIP

Another secret is the "hidden calorie burner." This consists of utilizing the power of low-impact exercises throughout your day. While taking the stairs to the third floor to go to work may seem insignificant, if you stack enough of these activities throughout the day, they will add up. Get in the mentality of adding in extra-credit workouts to your day-to-day activities, which may include:

- Taking the stairs.
- Parking further away.
- Ten-minute 'around the block' walks.
- Standing desks.

- Maxing out your grocery basket for that awesome shoulder workout!
- A quick stretch and mobility workout after waking up.
- Relying less on motorized transport for short distances.

Phase 5: Meal Timing (Intermittent Fasting)

Initially, I rejected things like intermittent fasting. I saw it as a fad, and worse, something that could throw your body into "starvation mode."

When I was first dieting, I didn't know what "starvation mode" was, but it sounded bad. I didn't want my body to hold onto every fat molecule with desperation, I wanted my body to throw caution to the wind and chuck the flub out the window.

I made sure my body was constantly fed to ward off the dastardly "starvation mode" state. This had me eating and snacking almost on an hourly basis since frequent small meals were the reigning method of dieting in my day. While I did lose weight, all those small meals and snacks took extra planning.

These days, things are different. I've educated myself and moved beyond concerns about losing muscle mass, starvation mode, and having crippling food cravings. I've adopted intermittent fasting into my lifestyle, and am thankful I did. You'll definitely want to learn about intermittent fasting too; some scientific studies show that it's a potent weight loss catalyst. For myself, it's a super simple way to maintain all that progress I've worked so hard for.

What is intermittent fasting? Simply put, intermittent fasting is not taking in calories for a set amount of time, regularly. Every day when we sleep for our six to ten hours, we are, in a manner of speaking, intermittent fasting. This is why we break the fast, with breakfast. Get it? Don't confuse this with starving yourself, or going super low-calorie. You're still trying to eat the same amount of calories that you would otherwise, they're just squeezed into a smaller feeding window.

When your body is in this fasted state, it makes hormonal changes that can stimulate your body to utilize your fat storage for energy. Insulin levels are lowered, insulin sensitivity is eventually increased, growth hormone levels are elevated (muscle preservation), and even our adrenaline levels (mental alertness) are increased after certain fasted periods. [18]

How long should you fast? There are tons of variations to intermittent fasting. The most popular seems to be the 16:8 schedule, where you basically have an eight-hour window to eat every day, and are fasting the other sixteen. With a sixteen-hour fast, you get a good balance between your sanity and the hormonal benefits described above. This is what I do, and it's as complicated as replacing breakfast with a hearty dose of black coffee (or your non-caloric beverage of choice), and eating between noon and eight. You can define your own schedule as you see fit, of course.

The 16:8 schedule may be the standard for most, but it's certainly not the only thing out there. You might see an extra hormonal benefit from reducing your feeding window further, or even going on twenty-four-hour to forty-eight-hour fasts from time to time. But if you're prone to binging behavior from cravings, it might not be the path yet. At the very least, it's something to think about, and possibly experiment with as a plateau buster.

Eventually, being more tolerant of time without food will help prevent slip-ups. I find that I don't get that "low blood sugar" feeling, or get ravenously hungry anymore. Because of this, I can calm the hunger signal which, at one time, might have led to poor decisions.

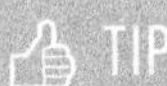

There are a lot of excellent resources freely available online to help one investigate the various facets of intermittent fasting. One I have used and recommend highly is:

- Reddit.com/r/IntermittentFasting/wiki/index

Phase 6: Count Them Calories

A time-tested way of taking off the pounds is by tracking everything down to the calorie. This is how the bodybuilders get super lean while being able to maintain their muscle mass and how I got through the last leg of my initial long-term goal of 9% body fat.

It's nearly bullet-proof, with a few caveats. Firstly, it won't work optimally if you're getting your calories from crap. Make sure you're eating well enough already, as outlined above. Secondly, some people have medical curveballs that might complicate the situation, so please confer with your health care team if appropriate.

I had already lost over 100 pounds before I ever needed (or wanted...) to micromanage my diet to the point of calorie counting, and I don't believe it to be of much use to the person just trying to get to a healthy weight and lead a better life.

> 👍 TIP
>
> CICO (calories in calories out, or calorie counting) is like a religion on the internet. There are a ton of people who adamantly believe it's the only way, and something you'll need to do for the rest of your life. Situations vary from person to person, but in my case, I've been able to utilize it to great benefit, and eventually trade it for what I believe to be an easier lifestyle. If you're wired for this kind of thing, you might love it. That's great! Do what's best for you. But if not, that's ok, know that there's a path for every personality.

With the information in this next section, I was able to transform myself from a healthy, normal weight (an admirable place to be) to totally lean. I utilized calorie counting to strike the final blow to the remaining fat mass, and achieve that sub 10% body fat goal I had set way back at the beginning of my journey. **If you are on the last leg of your transformation, if you've progressed through the previous phases of the plateau busting system, and if your eating habits are already dialed in, then calorie counting is for you.**

Starting with the basics, you need to know the three primary macronutrients. Your body uses proteins, carbohydrates, and fats to fuel its daily functions, which means everything from sitting on the couch, digesting food, to hiking mountains. Each one of these macronutrients has a calorie amount: proteins and carbohydrates have four calories per gram, and fat has nine. That's why one tablespoon of butter has significantly more calories than one tablespoon of honey.

What is a calorie? It's the baseline measurement of how much energy something gives you. The reason we have a jiggly belly is that we have been eating an excess (as well as the wrong kinds) of calories for a long enough time, this being our body's defense against times of famine. Our body hasn't evolved to realize that a power-packed meal costs six bucks down the road at Mickey D's, and that we can sit on our butts in front of a computer at work to make plenty of dough to cover that cost. It still thinks we have to hunt and forage for our food, and a dry season could be looming at any time.

Every day, just to exist, our body uses up calories just as a car would use up fuel, even if you turned it on and just left it sitting in park. This is known as our basal metabolic rate (BMR). It doesn't take into account the calories you use to change the channel or get up and grab an ice cream sandwich from the freezer. The BMR is just your body's calorie consumption as it sits, idling.

There isn't a really easy way to get the perfect estimate of your BMR because it depends on things such as genetics, metabolism, ambient temperature, and even how stressed out you are day-to-day. Metabolism has even been shown to take a huge nosedive if you've been crash dieting, as we've seen with the contestants of *The Biggest Loser*.[25] You can get an idea with the Harris-Benedict equation, just remember that these numbers are only rough estimates.

How to calculate your BMR (Harris-Benedict equation, revised version from 1990)[26]

Women's BMR

metric = (10 × weight in kg) + (6.25 × height in cm) - (5 × age in years) - 161

imperial = (4.536 × weight in pounds) + (15.88 × height in inches) - (5 × age) - 161

Men's BMR

metric = (10 × weight in kg) + (6.25 × height in cm) - (5 × age in years) + 5

imperial = (4.536 × weight in pounds) + (15.88 × height in inches) - (5 × age in years) + 5

So, let's say you take your car for a drive, or in human body terms, you do physical activity. This activity is calculated into your total daily energy expenditure (TDEE). The TDEE is your BMR plus any extra activities you do other than sitting there staring at the wall. The TDEE is more accurate than the BMR for calculating how much fuel (calories) it takes to run your body. This is an important number to know, because, quite simply, if you eat fewer calories than your TDEE (providing the caveats we discussed aren't hindering you), you'll lose weight, period.

Your body is not an anomaly that can transcend space and time, and it can't create its own energy. Although it may seem that we can sometimes defy the laws of physics, it's usually a miscalculation on our part. Your TDEE fluctuates from day-to-day, if you go to the gym it is higher, if you're catching up on *Seinfeld* reruns, it's lower.

How to calculate your TDEE

If you work at a desk job or are mostly sedentary = (BMR × 1.2)
If you exercise lightly 1-3 times a week = (BMR × 1.375)
If you exercise with moderate intensity 2-5 times a week = (BMR × 1.55)
If you are active most days = (BMR × 1.725)
If you have a very active job (construction) or are training every day multiple times a day = (BMR × 1.9)

However imprecise, this gives us a good starting point which we can tweak depending on the results.

Now, one pound of the chub on our belly is roughly 3,500 calories worth of energy, and if I use the example of my BMR from when I was 300 pounds, I use up about 2,375 calories just to count tiles in my ceiling in bed all day. If I want to shed 1 pound a week, I'd just have to figure out how many calories I need to cut each day to get to that goal. Let's do some math!

1 pound off the scale is equal to 3,500 fewer calories a week.

3500 divided by seven days equals 500, so to lose one pound a week I need to eat 500 fewer calories than my TDEE each day.

So, if I was lightly active (x1.375), the calories I would need to consume to just maintain my weight is 3,300, and eating 2,800 (3,300-500) calories a day would, technically speaking, give me a one pound a week weight loss.

Here is the math related to the above situation

BMR = (4.536 x 300(weight in pounds)) + (15.88 x 73(height in inches)) - (5 x 28(age)) +5 = 2,375

TDEE = (2,375 x 1.375) = 3,265 (let's average that to 3,300 to keep things simple)

3,300 minus 500 calories/day = 2,800 cals/day

So, if I eat 2,800 calories a day (as a 300 pound man that exercises lightly one to three days a week), I can expect (under perfect conditions) to lose about a pound a week.

Keeping track of your calories

food	carb	protein	fat	calories	servings		total carb	protein	fat	calories
							320	181	85	2144
1 large egg	0	6	5	70	6					
112g ground turkey	0	21	8	170	2					
1 avocado	1	1	27	276	0					
Isopure	0	40	0	160	0					
1 chobani pineapple yogurt	21	13	3	160	1					
Sunflower Seeds (100g)	24	19	50	582	0					
Wildflower meatball side	9	21	28	360	0					
carrots	21	12	3	35	5					
Salmon (100g)	0	20	13	208	0					
1 tbsp olive oil	0	0	14	119	0					
1 tbsp butter	0	0	12	200	0					
Banana	35	2	0	135	1					
Almonds (28g)	6	6	14	163	0					
1 large banana	35	2	0	135	0					
Oats (1/4 cup, 40g)	27	5	3	150	0					
1 cup chickpeas	36	12	4	220	0					
Rice & Lentils (100g)	22	6	0	114	3					

Now, you'll need a few things to start counting calories. First, to measure things, let's stop assuming and get a food scale and measuring cup, that way we can plug in the data as accurately as possible so we don't over- or under-shoot our calories.

You can track calories on paper, through a spreadsheet program, or utilize software or phone apps. It's easier than you think because your cell phone likely has a calorie counter already in it!

Samsung & Apple Health

This is likely the future of health monitoring because it is so all-inclusive. With my Samsung health application, I can take my pulse, check my blood oxygenation, track blood pressure, log my exercise with a GPS tracker, and of course, count calories. Technology is so sweet these days.

- Samsung.com/us/samsung-health/
- Apple.com/ios/health/

My Fitness Pal

A very popular program that I find wonderfully helpful is My Fitness Pal. It keeps tabs on your meals, snacks, and shows you how many proteins/carbs/fats you're eating, and even has a barcode scanner that utilizes your cell phone camera to help you keep track of things without having to plug in the data by hand. It's a fantastic resource, and probably much more advanced now than when this was written.

- Myfitnesspal.com/

Fit Bit

These little gizmos are all the rage these days, and fit on the wrist to help keep track of all sorts of interesting details, most notably your steps in the form of a pedometer. These days, the app is a bit more all-inclusive, and contains a calorie tracking section as well as a host of other interesting features. If you're not the type to lash out at inanimate objects telling you to get off your butt, this may be just the thing for you.

- Fitbit.com/app

Google Sheets

This is a spreadsheet program similar to Microsoft Excel which is free and perfectly capable of handling the job of keeping track of our calories. I preferred using a spreadsheet program like this back in the day to track my calories for maximum control. I set it up to help me decide each meal or snack to get in my macronutrient balance. This way is certainly more cumbersome, but it works!

- Google.com/sheets/about/

Count calories for a few days a week starting out, so that you're not overwhelmed by the increase in micromanagement. If you rely on your own staple foods list for the bulk of your eating, then calculating the calories is a lot easier. It gets hard when you try deconstructing the foods you get at a restaurant. P.S., they use more butter than you think.

It does feel annoying to have to do all this at first, but when you start seeing results, you'll know you've made the right choice. When you're ready, ramp it up to at least Monday-Friday, and adjust as you need.

If you aren't losing, take off 100 calories from the daily total, and try for another couple weeks. Pushing towards 9% body fat, I found that I didn't need to eat less than 2,200 calories to get the job done. If I went lower, I felt tired and my workouts suffered.

👍 TIP

Watch out for things with hidden calories. At one point early on, I was making Kool-Aid with Splenda thinking I had found a lovely little no-calorie loophole. I didn't even realize that when they say "no-calorie" sweetener, that they actually mean is "less than what the FDA requires to be documented as having calories," which just happens to be five calories per serving (each single-serving packet of Splenda has four calories, those sneaky bastards).

Long story short, I was drinking cups worth of Splenda per day, which was actually a significant amount of calories (upwards of 200 at times). Sometimes we forget to include these hidden calories. Here are a few items that really add up but that we don't always think about:

- Milk and sugar with coffee.
- Some types of chewing gum.
- Mints and candies.
- Oils and butter with cooking (fat isn't always bad, it's just high calorie).
- Mayo and other condiments.
- Don't get me started on salad dressings...
- High fructose corn syrup (or added sugars) in common food items.

Where should we get our calories from?

Protein intake is an important factor to take into account while dieting. One of the risks when starting things out is losing our muscle mass or fat-free mass (FFM). We want to preserve this stuff because it helps to increase our metabolism and keeps our body looking shapely after we lose that fat. This brings about the question: How much protein do we need anyway? This is a widely disputed question, and I have two ways to arrive at an acceptable amount.

Truth be told, we're not likely to have a protein deficit given our typically meat-centric culture these days. I'd love to add in piles of data and information suggesting specific protein ranges for those who are endurance athletes, powerlifters, and regular people, but for simplicity's sake, a well-regarded recommendation of 0.8 grams of protein per pound of FFM is a very reasonable protein goal for most of us. [27-31] This is not 0.8 grams of protein per the weight you see on the scale in the morning, but that weight minus the weight of fat mass from your body.

> **FFM** = Your current weight x (1 – body fat percentage in decimal format)

So, let's say I weigh 185 pounds, and I discovered my body fat percentage is 12, here is the math for that scenario.

$$185 \text{ x } (1 - .12) = 162.8$$

The FFM for the above example is 162.8, and I would need my FFM x 0.8 to arrive at my protein requirement to help maintain muscle mass during calorie restriction, which is around 130 grams of protein per day (162.8 x 0.8).

How do you discover your body fat percentage? You're more than welcome to go online and utilize a body fat percentage calculator to roughly determine the number, or use fancier methods (bod pod, skinfold caliper test, and bioelectrical impedance) for more accuracy. These more involved methods might be available in your area, and you can investigate with a Google search of "___ near me".

If you crave simplicity, like I do, there is an easier way that was recommended to me. While less precise, you can guestimate your ideal weight (or search online for "ideal weight calculator"); as a 6'1" reasonably muscular male, I'd like to think my ideal weight is around 170 to 180 pounds. 175 pounds (my rough ideal weight) x 0.8 = 140 grams of protein a day. This is similar to the previous amount (using FFM), and gives you an idea of how much protein you'll need.

Hitting the protein intake goal for the day will do a lot to help you preserve your muscle mass during calorie restriction (along with exercise). Make sure to fill the rest of your meals with tons of good, real food, and you'll be cruising.

Calorie counting isn't a perfect system, but it's one of the best ways to obtain maximum control over our diets. It's wonderful because it pushes us to look at how many calories everything has. For example, a Double Whopper is almost 1,000 calories. It'd take more than ten apples to get the same amount, or twelve pounds of celery. If you choose the right kinds of foods you'll be surprised by how filling your meals can be.

Don't be All-or-Nothing!

Danny Cahill steps on the scale and the numbers fluctuate for a moment. When they finally rest on 191, the crowd erupts. He raises his arms—the victory is his. He has lost a total of 239 pounds, over half his body weight, and the title to the winner of *The Biggest Loser*, Season 8, is his.

At that moment, this man exemplified the comeback. He stood basking in the glory of an epic win through the grueling physical and mental challenge of losing over a pound a day for 210 days.

But the story doesn't stop there. After winning $250,000, he continued this wave of positivity by speaking at numerous engagements, encouraging people to take hold of their lives.

Viewers across the world saw the stars align for this man, and his journey is a path that people want to follow.

It's common, when talking with friends and family in the throes of their own transformation, for them to go from no regulation to restrictions more fitting for bodybuilders in contest prep. This is known as the all-or-nothing transformation, and *The Biggest Loser* has people going from zero to breakneck speeds on day one.

Unfortunately, the majority of casual dieters fit this category, people who go from downtrodden and depressed to being swept up in a whirlwind of emotion and raw energy. WE WANT RESULTS!

I had a number of these all-or-nothing diet experiences, and they nerfed my self-confidence before I was actually able to make significant and lasting change.

At a certain point, the frustration boils over and then the pendulum swings to the opposite end. I had massive surges early on, where I ran every night, stopped eating all carbohydrates, weighed and measured everything, tried liquid diets, or other aggressively restrictive behaviors that inevitably led to the third stage in this process—lower self-esteem than I had before, and greater resentment. The cycle looks like this:

Frustration that boils over ➤ *aggressive attempts for progress* ➤ *burnout and a negative self-image*

This cycle is destructive. Successful long-term changes are gradual.

One study lends some clues as to why the all-or-nothing transformation doesn't work. Six years after the end of the competition, tests showed that Cahill's metabolism was significantly stunted.[32] In fact, they found this result in every single contestant they observed. We can suspect that the same happens to anyone who attempts the all-or-nothing transformation.

When you push your body to the brink, it pushes back. Cahill gained back over 100 pounds, but he's actually doing well compared to his reality-show teammates, who are mostly bigger than when they started. The experiment is a resounding failure.

You can tell that Cahill's intentions were to make something important through his struggle. His process reminds us that we must work with the body to obtain our goals and not fight against its underlying survival mechanisms.

Let's take a look at the regimen Cahill suffered through that pushed his body to reject the transformation:

Mr. Cahill set a goal of a 3,500-caloric deficit per day. The idea was to lose a pound a day. He quit his job as a land surveyor to do it.

His routine went like this: Wake up at 5 a.m. and run on a treadmill for forty-five minutes. Have breakfast— typically one egg and two egg whites, half a grapefruit and a piece of sprouted grain toast. Run on the treadmill for another forty-five minutes. Rest for forty minutes; bike ride nine miles to a gym. Work out for two and a half hours. Shower, ride home, eat lunch—typically a grilled skinless chicken breast, a cup of broccoli and ten spears of asparagus. Rest for an hour. Drive to the gym for another round of exercise.

If he had not burned enough calories to hit his goal, he went back to the gym after dinner to work out some more. At times, he found himself running around his neighborhood in the dark until his calorie-burn indicator reset to zero at midnight.[25]

It's masochistic to push yourself to these kinds of extremes. If you do, you could find yourself in the same boat, left with a body that is hell-bent on returning back to its former glory. How do you diagnose when you're in this regrettable situation? Here are a few warning signs:

- Harsh dietary restrictions followed by bingeing or epic blow-it days.
- Feeling like you're always dieting, yet are not making progress.
- Hating your diet, and fantasizing about quitting (discomfort is ok, not suffering).
- Large fluctuations in weight, or swings in emotion.
- January is diet month, February-December are anything goes months.

The all-or-nothing mentality also makes us prone to be excessively harsh with ourselves when mistakes are made. What's important is the mentality about messing up. When we expect them to happen, we aren't so surprised, and in turn, are less likely to have our ship capsized by them.

Mistakes can carry heavy guilt with them that leads to derailment—an unfortunate situation where slip-ups snowball out of control. To make meaningful progress, you aren't required to sell your soul to the transformation gods. Perfection is a silly ideology sold to us by advertising companies, so let's ditch the idea right now that this process will be totally smooth sailing.

"Failure is an event, never a person."

Make peace with your human qualities, with the fact that your transformation will not be perfect, that you will not always want to go to the gym, that you will slip up and eat a taco on a Tuesday now and then, that you will plateau… But if you go in knowing this, it won't defeat you. We are emotional beings, and forming new habits challenges our comfort level at times.

"Our greatest weakness lies in giving up. The most certain way to succeed is always to try just one more time."

👍 TIP

So, you made a mistake and ate something out of your plan. You might have had a major unplanned blow-it day. First of all, IT'S OK! Just take a moment to think about what happened. It might be helpful to break down the event as we discussed in the habit section. What was the cue, the routine, and the habit? **Write it down!** Make a plan for the next time a similar event happens.

Next, **don't try and undo the misstep**. On the very next day, continue on as if nothing had happened. Don't skip meals, and don't work out like a madman. Just keep moving forward. Also, you might want to skip a few days of stepping on the scale. You know what it's going to tell you anyway.

Putting It All Together

Food, once a source of frustration, is now fuel for the active and adventurous life I lead. Instead of occupying my thoughts, eating becomes just another part of the day, like checking my emails and brushing my teeth.

When I have a great meal, I still enjoy it immensely. I'm not like a cyborg absorbing food paste solely for nourishment. Food can be a drug, or it can be fuel. Work with it to turn the steering wheel in a direction that brings out the best in life.

Here is a short rundown of the most important details from this chapter:

- You don't have to give up the things you love.
- You don't have to adhere to strict eating habits perfectly, mistakes happen and it's ok.
- Eat real food, and eat a wide array of different foods.
- Develop your own food commandments, use my list as an example if you don't have a place to start.

- Try not to stuff yourself (Hara Hachi Bu), and eat mindfully.
- Prep meals so you can eat real food on the run and at work.
- Record what you eat for more control.
- Think about meal timing, and severely limiting sugars and other fast-digesting carbohydrates.
- Keep stepping up your fitness game, don't forget hidden calorie burners.
- Attack your food vices one by one.
- Count calories when you need maximum control.
- Ease into the challenges, don't be all or nothing!

Disclaimer

Desiring to make certain this information was not providing a disservice to those of you who are taking on your own transformation, I had a trained clinical expert and registered dietician offer critique. I understand that while the techniques I utilized in my own life worked wonderfully for me, it was my personal journey and might not work well for others. I was reassured with her approval and was encouraged to promote these tried and true principles.

However, one important note to mention was that if you have preexisting health concerns, such as diabetes or hormonal issues, you will want to have further input from your primary health care provider before you make drastic changes to your diet and lifestyle.

Please don't treat this as gospel, keep reading, learning, and developing your lifestyle. Every day we understand health and longevity more. Soon we'll have it all figured out, but until then, just do your best with the information you have.

FITNESS FOR LIFE

It can be automatic to associate the gym with pain and fitness boot camps and angry instructors setting grandiose and sadistic expectations. At this point, even a jog around the block might bring stabbing pains to the side of your stomach! I know the feeling...

There was a time when I felt like working out was just this annoying obligation: it's no fun but I gotta do it because, well, people say I should...What a lame reason. I knew it was lame, but I tried here and there, always inevitably sputtering myself out and feeling like a quitter when I rejected the idea of pushing myself to the brink again.

On the flipside, some people do love to workout. Are they brainwashed or are they gluttons for punishment? Is exercise something that eventually seems fun when you're doing it, but you just can't get past the hump of moving forward and it seems you need a pep talk to convince yourself every time?

We're all getting older. If we don't tell our bodies they need to move, we'll become more and more stuck. Eventually, making any progress might be like trying to stay afloat in a pool filled with pancake syrup.

Keeping our bodies strong and limber so we can live well now and in the future just makes too much sense.

Our bodies love to sweat and our hearts love to beat fast. It loves the sense of freedom that having strong lungs gives us, our face loves the open air, our animal side feels fulfilled when we lift weights and almost nothing is as peaceful as the feeling you get during the last five minutes of stillness in a tiring yoga session. Our social nature enjoys doing activities with other people; something we all know is good for us.

Sounds good on paper right? So what's the missing key towards unlocking that lifelong relationship with self-inflicted physical abuse?

Humble Beginnings

If you're like me when I was younger (I'm hoping not!), then physical education class is about the only consistent source of exercise you got. While there were times when I attempted sports, and played tag during recess, for the bulk of my teenage years I didn't go outside much and rather focused my attention on hand-eye coordination with my Nintendo consoles.

PE class was oftentimes a brutal lens that exposed my childhood inadequacies, and the rest of the kids knew it. If I didn't get picked last for some team sport, I felt pretty excellent.

Every year my school would do an assessment to see where we stood physically. This included push-up and sit-up tests. Imagine, if you will, the following scene: I was in the wrestling room with about thirty other kids and my best buddy at the time holding my feet as I tried to do as many sit-ups as I could within one minute.

Other than the huffing and puffing of a sea of kids, the most prominent sound was a massive fart I let out during my third sit-up. While my poor buddy held onto my feet, he looked away as if he was shielding his eyes from a recently detonated atomic bomb.

Thus began my own reputation as the gassy fat kid that I continually lived up to (you're welcome bully types who were searching for easy targets). Having that kind of reputation lingering over my head sealed my uncool fate.

One of the worst things about being a fat kid was anything related to endurance. While I had to commit to a physical education class, I was given a choice in junior high among a few different things. I took what I assumed to be the least strenuous one, weight lifting, and was quite dismayed when I discovered that we started each day with a lap around the quarter-mile track.

On day one, I couldn't even finish a lap at jogging pace, and had to walk at least half of it. Thankfully, the zombie apocalypse didn't happen then because I would have been the first course.

The weightlifting instructor was a man by the name of Coach Morgan. Bless him for being compassionate to me, because I really had some self-esteem issues in those days.

I caught a few giggles from the other kids as I lumbered into the weightlifting room last. Coach Morgan told them to shut it so forcefully that a vein on his brow looked like it was going to slap someone upside the head. This guy was buff as hell, and nobody crossed him. We got to the business of weightlifting, and since my muscles were well fed, I was rather strong by default.

Thinking back, I wasn't made fun of much in weightlifting class, even when Coach Morgan wasn't hovering around us. We were all there to get stronger and better ourselves. Every weekday, I'd show up, attempt the lap, and go through various routines including chest, back, and legs. Every week I got stronger. Within a few months, I was able to conquer the lap at a gingerly jogging pace, which was a pretty cool accomplishment at the time.

The "I Can" Plan

I first realized the idea of "I can" through fitness. Through this lens, improvement feels more visceral, and changes happen quickly. While ten pounds on a scale might be almost unnoticeable when you look in the mirror, accomplishing some random fitness goal feels awesome. Your body knows things are going well too and will reward your hard efforts with a myriad of benefits.

Towards the end of my time in Coach Morgan's weightlifting class, I was benching over 100 pounds and feeling better about myself. Through the years, achieving certain benchmarks in fitness have been some of the most rewarding things I've experienced in my whole life. Maybe it sounds a bit over the top, but the snowball effect kept building upon itself until I was capable enough to do all sorts of things.

I didn't know what to expect by rebuilding my body. I had hoped, of course, that I would lose weight, become healthy, and maybe impress a couple of girls in the process. I didn't expect how much the doors of the world would swing open for me. The same happens for everybody who goes through this kind of transformation.

It's scientifically possible to lose every ounce of your extra weight through diet alone. When people say this to me however, I cringe. So many people will casually mention that diet is 80% and exercise is 20%, but I think they're missing the point. I wouldn't have even been inspired to go to these lengths in my life were it not for the world that the active life showed me.

You might not want to summit Mount Everest, or run a marathon, but if you aren't sweating a bit now and then, you may very well be missing out on life-changing inspiration. I know with absolute certainty that I would have.

Getting Over the Hump

Getting over the hump is tough. The first wave of motivation comes, you get to it, but repeating the same ass kicking over and over gets hard. If it hurts like hell every time, then only someone of superhuman willpower can keep it up.

Here's the thing, I'm definitely not one of those people, and you don't have to be one either to get results.

When you see the best athletes in the world training for the big day, it's only the most intense-looking training that we witness. We don't see their mellow workouts which likely make up the majority of their day-to-day.

We can build up in our minds that the requirements of our transformation are going to be beyond our ability, and in suggesting it, think it's "just not for me." Truth is, most of what it took for me to get muscular was actually relaxing, and all of it was fun. I wouldn't have gotten so far if it wasn't, because I need to emphasize again, I'm not one of those people.

There's a nifty little concept called "Flow" as popularized by a guy named Mihaly Csikszentmihalyi (don't ask me to pronounce that). He wrote a book describing an optimal growth state that can conveniently be applied to about a million things. For our purposes, let's summarize the idea by suggesting that there is this happy place between working out balls to the wall, and wishing you were somewhere else trotting on a treadmill.

This is the flow channel, or the right level of challenge so that you're not stressed out or bored. It's the optimal area for performance, growth, etc. Most importantly, it's how to make exercise enjoyable.[33]

I'd love to talk about all of my failed attempts at becoming a regular with exercise, but I'm sure you've probably heard it all before (or lived it). A lot of the stories begin with a fit friend casually inviting me to do a random fitness class with them. What for them was an everyday experience, was an absolute earth-shattering ass kicking for me. I tell them how much fun I had while hiding the resentment for the week of pain I know will follow. Our schedules just never seemed to work out after that...They were in the flow channel, while I was in a state of heavy stress trying to keep up.

Instead of these infrequent earth-shattering ass kickings, I found a happy place with fitness by staying in my own flow channel. When I started to get to a mental state where

I wasn't having fun, or feeling too much pain, I changed the pace to get into the flow.

The reality of the situation is that I became better trained and actually wanted to train more by being less of a hardass on myself. Then, when the mood strikes me, I'll go all out for some physical challenge and have fun doing it. It's nice to know what your body can do, but you'll never discover it by going all out every time.

Athletic coach Firas Zahabi says "I'm a firm believer in consistency over intensity."[34] By going through the motions, and finding that happy place in the flow channel, you'll be heading in the direction of a healthy addiction with fitness.

A Lazy Dog Whines, a Happy Dog Plays

Once, while traveling in Mexico, I happened upon a large indoor food market. One thing I'll never forget about the experience was one of the most incredibly fat dogs I've ever seen. This thing was an absolute unit and looked exhausted to just exist.

The poor bastard sat there and heaved with each breath as he waited for snacks from the passersby. He looked nothing like the lean, ancestral animal that he was bred from. Even though I was unaware of his inner doggie thoughts, he looked unhappy, and lacked every ounce of energy his pup buddies seemed to have endless amounts of. This really made me think about my fellow humans, and how I was similarly once this sad, obese kid.

Our brains are basically a modded version of the monkey brains of our ancestors. Within the mechanics of our mind is a circuit which, when stimulated with exercise and play, produces a myriad of psychological benefits. When it hasn't been stimulated, I imagine the animal inside our mind to start looking more like the huge overweight doggie.

It may seem silly for an adult to play, but if you think about it, it's silly for us *not* to play. We play throughout our youth, and tend to phase it out as we grow older so we can make time for all that crap that comes with being a well-adjusted adult. If you shuddered at the last sentence, there's hope for you yet.

Dr. Stuart Brown heads an organization called the National Institute for Play (sounds so official) and describes play as "Something done for its own sake. It's voluntary, it's pleasurable, it offers a sense of engagement, it takes you out of time. And the act itself is more important than the outcome."[35]

If you're breaking a sweat while you're playing, it doesn't feel like exercise, and that's another secret for making working out fun. To a kid though, this is no secret. Playing is a way of life.

When I was in elementary school, we had a student council. God knows what any of these kids really did, and how a twelve year old was supposed to be constructive in any position of power. I wasn't a part of this, but I remember that the class president, Robbie, handily took the throne with a singular platform on adding more recess.

He didn't make much sense and mumbled through half of the speech, but the auditorium erupted when he said he'd add more recess. How can you not vote for that?! I certainly wasn't going to be that one guy to vote for the other dorks suggesting that the textbooks be updated.

Did we get our second recess, hell no, twelve-year-olds have no political sway and we hated Robbie for it. We exacted sweet revenge on him because of this failed presidency. My pals and I devised a sabotage plot to sneakily attach a "Sex Educator" pin we found in a parking lot to his backpack. Soon after that stunt though he acquired a girlfriend. In hindsight I wonder if we ended up helping him out...

Truth is, Robbie's ideas weren't crazy. He just wanted an escape from the grind like the rest of us. Kids already know the things us adults have to pay therapists tons of cash to tell us. They know that getting outside, chilling with your buds, moving around, and playing are all good things.

If kids don't get a chance to play, they fidget more, eat more junk food, and have lower test scores. [36].

Do you think it's any different for adults? It's even more magnified. You want to deprive a human of play, well the consequences include:

- Depression.
- Compulsive behavior.
- Diminished optimism.
- Sense of being a victim as opposed to a winner.
- Decrease in effectiveness across the board. [35]

How the heck is anybody supposed to accomplish anything with those feelings coursing through their mind?

Half of the time, I feel like that kid anxiously looking at the clock waiting for recess. When I incorporate some play into my every day, I feel better, more capable, and more content. And because my play is also my way to get exercise, it's a win-win.

Forget what kind of things you "should" be doing, because if you're having fun you don't have to pep talk yourself off that recliner with the built in cup holders. I could get crazy eyes gushing about the benefits of lifting weights, but if you're easily offended by body odor, hanging out in a rusty gym dungeon might not work.

What *does* work is realizing that you don't have to trot on a treadmill until your head implodes from boredom. If fitness isn't your thing, that means you're doing the wrong activities, so be open to new experiences and keep trying.

👍 TIP

If you really want to do something fun, try training for an event or local competition of some kind. You don't even have to participate in it because they're fun to watch! You'd be hard pressed to find a more positive and supportive crowd than those in fitness circles. Check your local sports stores, the newspaper, or the Internet for events happening in your area. You can try:

- Hiking clubs.
- Zumba or outdoor yoga classes.
- Weightlifting meets or bodybuilding competitions.
- Mud runs or obstacle courses.
- 5ks, triathlons, half marathons etc…

While it's important to have fun with your fitness, relying on fun every time might make it hard to exercise when the opportunities aren't available for the things you like to do. At these times it's really important to have a few back-up ideas under your belt if you find yourself unable to participate in your normal activities.

As reluctant as I always have been towards running, I've found that being able to run a few miles makes it easy to exercise almost anywhere. Beyond that, a basic calisthenics routine (using your own bodyweight to workout) will go a long way in keeping you fit even if you were stuck in a jail cell.

What's the Endgame?

If you've ever met someone that diets in obviously bad ways, you'll know how tortured they look. I once heard of a woman who lived for months on a diet of cigarettes and Monster energy drinks. Her body withered away to the point where she could fit nicely in those skinny jeans, but the tanning booth couldn't bring life back into her grey skin. She also wasn't very friendly, but how could she be? If your body is pissed off, you'll be pissed off too.

If you ever go onto social weight loss forums or reddit, you'll see countless posts that are some version of this:

> *"Is it possible to lose thirty*
> *pounds in the next week?"*

The responses range the gamut, but thankfully some do try to impart a bit of rational thinking on the hurried poster. (Maybe recommend the Monster energy drink and cigarette diet?)

What's the common thread between these people? They're thinking way too short-term. Now, before I start sounding like an ancient philosopher who has it all figured out, let me correct that idea right away. I too am majorly guilty of thinking short-term to the detriment of my own body. I wish it weren't so, because I could have happily avoided a few injuries.

What's the timeline in your goals? By this point, I'm hoping you've given some thought to a long-term and short-term goal, but what about way down the road? We're talking ten years from now, maybe even into retirement. Isn't that important too?

It's hard to think that far ahead, and oftentimes I did not during my own transformation. I eventually realized that setting myself up for the future is the best plan. We all need to think about our own endgame.

Here's a simple thought exercise: Imagine you end up living a long life, and luck out with all the "hold my beer and watch this" moments between now and retirement age. How can you set up the old-fart version of you so that you can look proudly on these days spent transforming yourself, instead of shaking your head and muttering, "you young, hot-headed fool!"

Have you ever heard of Ronnie Coleman? This guy is one of the most astoundingly huge Mr. Olympias and at the time of writing this ties Lee Haney for most wins of all time at eight. He gave everything for his physique, even his health.

If you watch the documentary *Ronnie Coleman: The King*, you'll see a man ravaged by years of brutal training, who pops the maximum prescribable dose of Oxycodone like Tic-Tacs to deal with his chronic pain. He will go down in history as one of the greatest bodybuilders of all time, but I can't help being saddened by his current plight. He pretty much gave up his future health for the glory of his accomplishment, because he trained harder than anybody.

Now, I don't want to discredit his amazing accomplishments, but I know that within some of us is a piece of that fire that he has. This fire rages hot when we get caught up in the moment, and when those veins start bulging like we're in berserker mode. Training to be the best in the world is one thing, but if you're trying to be your best, think about that old timer down the road.

Here are a few suggestions to help us age gracefully while also keeping fit:

Warm up Gently

Take time easing into the motions of exercise; go for a short walk or slow jog before you run, do some lightweight reps before you start stacking on the pounds. Get your joints used to the motion before they're suddenly shocked. A standard routine might look like this:

1. Warm your body up with some basic aerobic exercise.

2. Actively mobilize your joints using the range of motion you expect to do. "For runners, that might mean high knees, butt kicks, walking lunges, and side skips."[37]

3. Ease into the actual exercise, going at a moderate starting pace (or weight) and ramping it up until you reach your goal.

Balance Your Exercises

Focusing on one thing will lead to imbalances in your muscle development. It's good to focus, but make sure to balance it out with inverse exercises to prevent misalignment; if you want a huge chest, work your back too, if you want to run really far, do resistance training with your legs too.

This is why trainers recommend cross training, or in other words, doing different stuff now and then so your muscles get exercised in different ways. Balance is key.

Make Mobility and Stretching a Daily Habit

Flexibility will leave your body faster than you realize, something I'm learning as I pass my mid-thirties. But you don't have to cripple yourself with stiff joints if mobility is part of the plan.

Interestingly, there are plenty of scientists searching for the illusive benefits of static stretching (you know, touching your toes and that kind of thing), and their association to injury avoidance.[37]

Regardless of the evidence, I can say for certain that picking stuff off the ground, squeezing into cheap airplane seats, and scratching my back are all easier with a little bit of flexibility. Stretching is a really enjoyable part of the routine too. After I've had a good sweat, slowing down the pace with a relaxing stretching session caps things off nicely. Plus, after your muscles have had time to warm up, they're more pliable and take to a good stretch better. If you want a good functional routine, just go to a yoga class, they have it figured out.

Listen to Your Body (Don't Push Through Pain)

When I rewind to my time learning to lift weights, it's punctuated by injury. The injuries happened because I wasn't listening to my body. I was lifting weight that caused my form to suffer, and pushing through pain when I should have been resting.

Some of these injuries cause me chronic pain to this day, years later, a theme which seems to be all too familiar with older friends of mine. One mentioned, after a very serious surgery to repair damaged vertebrae in his neck, "I wish I had picked up yoga in my twenties instead of lifting like I was in a Rocky montage all the time." You don't have to experience the same fate.

Form is way more important than the poundage. Stop trying to be a badass and remember that it doesn't count if you're cheating your way to the end of the rep (I'm looking at you Crossfit). Keep an eye on yourself when you're doing your exercises, gym mirrors are helpful for this, or better yet get a qualified trainer to keep your form in check.

The Active Life is Best

When you have a healthy relationship with fitness, you will find that many of the challenges that come along with the transformation shrink. Exercise helps on multiple fronts, from burning fat and building strength, to burning stress and building confidence.

Instead of me telling you what's best, just learn to develop a relationship with an increased heart rate and sweat. Really, who cares how it's done (so long as it's not robbing banks!). This story is different for everybody involved.

Fitness, to me, has become less an "activity" that I do, and much more a way of life, a part of me. As silly as it sounds, I truly believe that the gym and the hiking trails are sacred places. Without this curious exploration of my own comfort zone, I might have never experienced some of my most cherished things, from meeting my wife, to adventures while traveling all over the globe. You should definitely not miss out on this opportunity for inspiration, for kinship, and for health.

BECOME A MASTER OF MOTIVATION

> "Wanting something is not enough. You must hunger for it. Your motivation must be absolutely compelling in order to overcome the obstacles that will invariably come your way."
>
> LES BROWN, AMERICAN MOTIVATIONAL SPEAKER AND AUTHOR

The movie ends and the credits begin. You sit there in silence in a whirlwind of thought. *This* is exactly what I needed, you think, my soul is alive.

And so it begins, tomorrow is the day it changes... Epiphanies blossom in your mind. I'm going to ask that girl out, I'm going to run a mile, I'm going to tell my boss I've had enough! You hardly sleep because your mind is calculating away. The odds may be stacked against you, but it's now or never.

Sleep eventually comes, and morning limps in. Where there was once power, there is now vulnerability. Motivation, previously cruising on rocket fuel, is now running on its backup tank of used restaurant peanut oil, sputtering like an old car.

What happened? Motivation came and went. The sinking feeling of reality stamped it out.

Motivation is such a strong word. In seeking to cultivate it, there are motivational videos, books, artwork with majestic mountains and thought-provoking quotes, as well as those epic speakers that stoke audiences to sheer ecstasy.

Motivation is seen as a key component of the transformation. "If only I had the motivation to change," you might say. And so we spend our efforts trying to discover the missing puzzle piece.

The most accomplished people seem fueled by incredible motivation; these are our athletes, business owners, professionals, and high-caliber people of every kind. The world watches them in awe, wondering what lessons can be gleaned from their minds. Understanding this motivation has been a personal quest of mine as well.

I sought the silver bullet, that drop of wisdom to unlock my maximal motivational potential. This brought me to the tutelage of some powerhouse human beings and left me to face some hard truths.

Motivational Psychology

When we think about motivation, it's like this magical force that levitates our butts off the couch. My inner voice would often ask, "why do I feel so energized sometimes, and how can I feel this more often?"

When you recall times of surged energy, what clues lay within the mists to identify the source of this elusive motivational power? I'm willing to bet that while you know you *felt* good, it might not be so easy to explain why.

Where do those who succeed with their own transformations find this motivation, and is it a lack of motivation that causes someone to become overweight in the first place? Well, there are a few people I'd like to introduce you to. Maybe they can help shed some light on this motivation stuff.

I'll start by introducing you to Brian. He's the dude we want hanging around us all the time. With Brian, you get things done. Brian compliments you when he sees you, he's able to tell you about his plans and describe them so energetically that it seems foolish not to tag along. He's a *force of nature*. This person has a goal, and the drive to accomplish them. Brian is pretty much a badass, and regardless of what you're up to, things will get better when he's along for the ride.

Then we have Alex, he's not a bad guy, but people don't get too carried away when they tell stories about him. Not like that Brian guy, what a character! But Alex ain't a bad guy, he's doing okay in his life and he has a few cool goals lingering around. We know he has a few goals because he talks about them from time to time, although he doesn't seem to be making much headway. Brian and Alex have always been pals, but Brian is always occupied with something and isn't available to get on Alex's case about his goals. When they get together though, Alex can't help but rekindle his dreams, if only for a short while.

Truth is, Alex's in a rut. He can't help but wonder what his future could look like under different circumstances, like perhaps if Brian were around more often to whip him into shape. Brian is going places, man, and Alex is just going through the motions. Alex hasn't forgotten about his dreams though.

Brian shouldn't have to hold Alex's hand and guide him to his dreams. Alex has got to create his own fate. It's awesome having Brian as a resource, as an energizing shot of Red Bull now and then, but what if Brian isn't around? Should Alex just throw up his hands and toss in the towel?

That's the first thing about understanding motivation. We've all got our own Brian and Alex inside of us. When our emotions are peaking, when we're inexplicably feeling good, Brian is paying us a visit. We're human after all, and there's a lot of hormonal, environmental, and psychological reasons for our unpredictable emotions. Sometimes Brian is there, but usually, he isn't. Brian, while motivating, is not true motivational power. Don't mistake one for the other.

Our emotional power (Brian) is unpredictable and unreliable. True motivation comes from somewhere else. So, where is this alternate energy source?

When psychologists talk about motivation, they break it down into two categories: extrinsic and intrinsic.[38] In short, extrinsic motivation is all about those things seen as beneficial side effects to the accomplishment of your goals, be it money, fame, notoriety, and so forth. These motivational factors are indeed powerful, as some of the most capable and driven athletes are no doubt pushed by the financial benefits of their performance.

Wouldn't it be sweet to get paid millions of dollars to focus on weight loss? Hell, I'd bet that would motivate almost anybody to get the job done. Unfortunately, unless you're a contestant on *The Biggest Loser*, I doubt you're getting paid a penny. Here are a few other extrinsic motivators that did have some influence over me:

- Desire to be attractive to women. (Chicks man...)
- Displeasure with being seen by others as a failure.
- Embarrassment in public situations that highlighted my weight issues.
- Desire to look good in clothing.

These cheesy influences will only get you so far, but there's limitless energy somewhere else. This is the coveted intrinsic motivation, and studies have found that those who are driven by their internal flame show way stronger determination over the long run.[39]

> "Often children—and adults—need external incentives to take the first steps in an activity that requires a difficult restructuring of attention. Most enjoyable activities are not natural; they demand an effort that initially one is reluctant to make. But once the interaction starts to provide feedback to the person's skills, it usually begins to be intrinsically rewarding"
>
> MIHALY CSIKSZENTMIHALYI,
> QTD. IN "FLOW: THE PSYCHOLOGY OF OPTIMAL EXPERIENCE"

So, what's the double barreled shotgun for your motivation arsenal? How can you work towards that nuclear-powered internal flame? I have a few recommendations; they're called the **Mandates of Motivation™**.

Mandates of Motivation

Mandate 1: Don't Rely on Being Motivated

We spent some time talking about Brian and Alex, and how Alex needs to learn to take care of business on his own terms. The thing is, motivation will fail you eventually. When you feel good, motivation keeps you focused, but what about when you aren't feeling it? What then?

You know more than enough to get started, but if you're goofing off and winging it, you're relying on wishy-washy emotions to fuel your pushes instead of a plan.

You won't genuinely fix anything until the underlying machinery for success that lies behind the transformation is established, and the base levels are your goals and plans. Once you have these, and once you're committed, you won't have to pray for motivation. You just follow the path you've set.

> "Better to cultivate discipline than to rely on motivation. Force yourself to do things. Force yourself to get up out of bed and practice. Force yourself to work. Motivation is fleeting and it's easy to rely on because it requires no concentrated effort to get. Motivation comes to you, and you don't have to chase after it.

Discipline is reliable, motivation is fleeting. The question isn't how to keep yourself motivated. It's how to train yourself to work without it."

ANONYMOUS

Mandate 2: Define Your Purpose

Deep in the recesses of your identity lies something powerful. Maybe our soul defines it, or maybe personalities from past lives are whispering to us, who knows. I do know one thing, though: when you live for a purpose, when you act on behalf of something great, new strength will overcome you.

I recently happened upon a video of a child asking Richard Dawkins, an ethologist, evolutionary biologist, and author, what he thought was the purpose of life. After pondering the question, he responded with a perplexing rationale for human purpose that is worthy of consideration.

In the video, Dawkins talks about how we're in a fortunate position as a species where we almost never have to worry about basic human needs like food, water, and shelter. Even those without homes can be reasonably assured aid exists somewhere. We truly live in amazing times.

While moving beyond these struggles is a major reason for the improvement in the lives of humankind across the globe, it has muddled our purpose. This leads us to widespread existential dilemmas. Freedom of choice is confusing. With our needs met, what are we to do now? Have we, through technology, industrialization, and agriculture replaced the notion of a purpose with a nine-to-five job? Hardly!

When Dawkins responded, he observed that, given our new freedoms, we must define our own purpose. The meaning of our lives lies within the depths of our imagination.

Knowing what we want means an incredible amount. It gives us a point to work towards. This is exactly why the first step I outlined is defining a vision. We must see ourselves forged into all the good things we idealize so that we have something to work towards.

Now that you have a what, decide your own why. I saw the direction I was headed in and observed what I was passionate about. Even if I hadn't labeled it, my purpose was already expressing itself in my actions.

When I took the time to observe this purpose, and write it down, I started doing more things that supported it, while less important things took a backseat.

This book is one facet of the purpose I defined. After years of struggle and finally breaching rough waters, I unconsciously acted towards writing down my own process. I'd always thought that if I could beat my sickness, I should help others through it as well. I have found that acting for others, for something greater than myself, keeps me from giving up during the long haul.

"The most important trait of survivors is a 'nonself-conscious individualism,' or a strongly directed purpose that is not self-seeking. People who have that quality are bent on doing their best in all circumstances, yet they are not concerned primarily with advancing their own interests."

MIHALY CSIKSZENTMIHALYI
QTD. IN "FLOW: THE PSYCHOLOGY OF OPTIMAL EXPERIENCE"

✍ WRITE IT DOWN

Think hard about the things that fill you with hope and excitement. Ponder your own purpose. A purpose need not be only one thing. It certainly wasn't for me. It should be more abstract than a specific goal—think big picture. Tonight, or as soon as you can, create a purpose statement. I've included some sample purpose statements that you're free to use as a blueprint for your own.

My life purpose is to (a few ideas):

- Develop mastery of myself and conquer my health problems.
- Become the best version of myself for my wife/child/parents/dog.
- Encourage others struggling with their own weight issues.
- (You may find strength in a spiritual pursuit here.)

We started with a vision, created goals, action plans, and now purpose statements. What it all boils down to is living deliberately, that is, understanding what we want, why we want it, and how we're going to get it.

With a strong purpose, we'll have a brick wall to lean on when scrounging for motivation is hard. I've found that in times of confusion and turmoil, the purpose I've created keeps me moving.

Mandate 3: Reduce Your Life Stressors

During my time at university one of my professors had our class take a survey. Out of curiosity, she had decided to see how much the stress we were dealing with in our personal lives related to our test scores.

The survey was based on research done in the 1960s by psychiatrists Thomas Holmes and Richard Rahe.[40] The question they posed was whether illness could be correlated with stressful life events.

This questionnaire added up various life events and their related "life-changing units" to provide a total stress score. This was then given to patients in a hospital setting and statistically analyzed to assess health outcomes and their relation to these stressors.

They discovered that the test was not only a reliable predictor of health outcomes, but things such as academic success and employee absenteeism. Interestingly, there ended up also being a strong correlation between elevated stress scores and lower test scores in my class.

Stress stacks, and very much affects our ability to sustain motivation. Because of this, some people are at a higher predisposition to face trouble in their own transformations. Take a look below and see where you fall on the spectrum of stress.

<table>
<tr><td colspan="2" align="center">The Holmes and Rahe Stress Scale</td></tr>
<tr><td>

1. Death of a spouse **100**
2. Divorce **73**
3. Marital Separation **65**
4. Jail term **63**
5. Death of a close family member **63**
6. Personal injury or illness **53**
7. Marriage **50**
8. Fired at work **47**
9. Marital reconciliation **45**
10. Retirement **45**
11. Change in health of family member **44**
12. Pregnancy **40**
13. Sex difficulties **39**
14. Gain of a new family member **39**
15. Business readjustments **39**
16. Change in financial state **38**
17. Death of a close friend **37**
18. Change to different line of work **36**
19. Change in # of arguments with spouse **35**
20. Mortgage over $50,000 **31**
21. Foreclosure of mortgage **30**
22. Change in responsibilities at work **29**

</td><td>

23. Son or daughter leaving home **29**
24. Trouble with in-laws **29**
25. Outstanding Personal achievements **28**
26. Wife begins or stops work **26**
27. Begin or end school **26**
28. Change in living conditions **25**
29. Revision of personal habits **24**
30. Trouble with boss **23**
31. Change in work hours or conditions **20**
32. Change in residence **20**
33. Change in school **20**
34. Change in recreation **19**
35. Change in religious activities **19**
36. Change in social activities **18**
37. Loan less than $50,000 **17**
38. Change in sleeping habits **16**
39. Change in number of family get-togethers **15**
40. Change in eating habits **15**
41. Vacation **13**
42. Holidays **12**
43. Minor violation of laws **11**

</td></tr>
</table>

- Each event should be considered if it has taken place in the last twelve months. Use the values denoted in bold to the right of each item. When finished, add the values to obtain your total score.

- Here is your susceptibility to illness and mental health problems (or even troubles with your transformation):

Low < 149	Mild 150—200
Moderate 200—299	Major >300

It's important to realize how much our motivation can be stifled by stress. It's safe to say that our ability to manage or reduce these stresses will determine our ability to stay focused on this quest of transformation.

Mandate 4: Willpower Fuel

Think of willpower as if it were a tank of fuel that refills every night when we get some solid sleep. When the day is young and your tank is full, you're ready to take on any challenge. The more filled up your willpower tank is, the easier things seem. Conversely, when your tank is low, it might even be hard to get up from the couch. Being aware of our willpower tank is helpful, and being productive before it's tapped out is crucial.

> "If you want to do something that requires willpower—like going for a run after work—you have to conserve your willpower muscle during the day... If you use it up too early on tedious tasks like writing emails or filling out complicated and boring expense forms, all the strength will be gone by the time you get home."
>
> *MARK MURAVEN,*
> *QTD. IN "THE POWER OF HABIT" BY CHARLES DUHIGG*

Think about your day; think about the times when it's hardest to make the right choices. Sometimes, by reorganizing tasks, you can plan accordingly to optimize their draining effects on motivational fuel. This is one of the reasons why people find exercising in the morning so beneficial.

Nothing beats waking up and hitting a productive stride in the morning. Though many have a concept of the ideal morning routine, I find that, in practice, it's not always easy to adhere to. Our lives have lots of variables from day-to-day. That's ok, but here are some recommendations that I do my best to follow.

- Practice good sleep hygiene the night before.
- Don't be in a rush in the mornings, wake up earlier if you have to.
- Review goals and plans for the day.
- Drink a tall glass of water.
- Do something physical, even if it's just for a few minutes (a few bodyweight squats to loosen the hips).
- Do things in the morning that require the most will-power energy or conserve your fuel until you need it.
- Meditate if that's a part of your practice.

Tim Ferriss, an entrepreneur and author of several self-help books including *The 4-Hour Work Week*, recommends keeping your phone on airplane mode so that you don't wake up with a pile of notifications and "short circuit" your morning.

I find that my most productive days follow a good morning routine.

Mandate 5: Team Up!

> "Associate with those who will make a better man of you. Welcome those whom you yourself can improve. The process is mutual; for men learn while they teach."
>
>

Some of us have to contend with our own transformations as a solo venture. This was largely my personal situation. I became fond of going to the deserted apartment complex gym (photographed here) where my love of fitness truly blossomed. It's important that you build this relationship with yourself and your goals, and that you nurture this venture so that you're not dependent on outside resources.

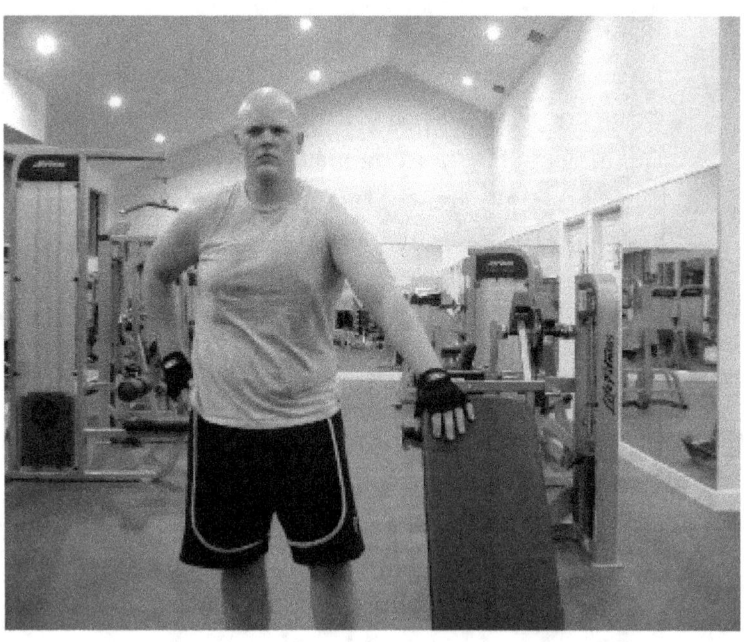

However, the final surge to my first long-term goal of reaching 9% body fat was definitely strengthened by having someone to be accountable to. I had an excellent teammate with whom I became competitive. We made some strict goals that ended up swiftly kicking the ass of my remaining fat. Here were the big ones:

- No added sugar in any form (fruit was OK).
- No artificial sweeteners of any kind (No Diet Mountain Dew...my last vice!)
- No milk or milk products.
- 4 liters of water a day, minimum.

I had already been tracking my food in a spreadsheet log, calorie counting, and catering my diet to match a specific macronutrient ratio. Adding the above to the list really made my lifestyle restrictive!

The amazing thing about it was that I managed to adhere to it perfectly. While, at this point, my own drive was burning brightly, the added concern of potentially faltering in front of my teammate was unacceptable. I learned how helpful it was to have someone working with me on collective goals. Even when I didn't have her breathing down my neck, I was still determined to stick to it.

"There's something really powerful about groups and shared experiences. People might be skeptical about their ability to change if they're by themselves, but a group will convince them to suspend disbelief. A community creates belief."

Stanford psychologists have studied this phenomenon, and it holds weight. Psychologist Gregory Walton stated, "That simply feeling like you're part of a team of people working on a task makes people more motivated as they take on challenges."[41]

So, it may be beneficial to seek out a buddy to hold you accountable to the demands of your transformation. Significant others, friends and family members definitely constitute a great place to start, as it makes it easier to confide your challenges in them. But don't discount seeking accountability buddies online; there are many places where people in your same exact situation can be found. Some find it helpful to write their diet logs in forum posts, where, instead of personal contacts, strangers can help you through these challenges. Don't dismiss any of these opportunities to aid you in your mission!

Another type of buddy I have benefited greatly from is a mentor. Becoming a regular at the gym can be beneficial in this way, and I lucked out with a competitive bodybuilder who was happy to take me under his wing. This dude, even in his fifties, was still entering bodybuilding competitions. He had been through it all, and though he's compensated well for the advice that he dishes out to his customers, he managed to get my head on straight with the new challenges

I faced simply by seeing my eagerness to learn and realizing my work ethic.

Throughout my transformation, I've come across many people who were gracious with their knowledge and experience. This is partly why I adore fitness circles as much as I do.

Here are some excellent places to meet like-minded people:

Local groups

WW International (Weight Watchers): I wholeheartedly approve of this organization. Although it's not free, the cost of membership is reasonable (less than a buck a day at the time of writing), and it includes a community of individuals who are there to support you through your transformation and who are also on their own journey. While it started as a women's group, it has opened its doors today to both sexes, so don't be a tough guy. Check it out:

- Weightwatchers.com/us/find-a-meeting/

Meetup.com: This website is a collection of individuals who aim to start up local clubs and organizations of all kinds. A great many have used it to start their own weight loss support groups. It's free to use and usually the groups are free too, unless the organizer has specified otherwise. Take a peek and see if there's a group meeting near you!

- Meetup.com/

Internet communities

Reddit.com: Reddit is a wonderful and potentially dangerous website where people go to post any number of things.
It's easy to waste an afternoon on this website (I'm guilty as
charged), so beware. It's also wonderful in the sense of it
being a place where people go to connect with each other,
chat, and troubleshoot their lives. I'm a member of one of
these communities (you can browse without signing up)
called /r/loseit, that I find to be a great resource for successful dieters. For fitness advice, check out /r/fitness.

- Reddit.com/r/loseit/
- Reddit.com/r/fitness/

Bodybuilding.com: Don't let the name fool you. This
website doesn't just cater to bodybuilders. This community helped me learn and develop as I was starting out with
weight loss. I absolutely adore their setup. Not only is the
community strong, but the tracking tools are awesome and
include graphs to show visuals of your weight, measurements, and lifts. The people here were very supportive and
always ready to lift me up when I was down. Check it out,
it's free:

- Forum.bodybuilding.com/forumdisplay.php?f=16

You can also start your own community in the workplace
or among friends. **Your opportunity for success with the
transformation only improves by being part of a team, so
do yourself a favor and get involved.**

On the flip side, while teammates are wonderful, depending on our teammates too much can set us up for trouble. I

remember long ago a family member dear to me went to the hospital for major surgery. Since the surgery took place in Arizona where I was living at the time, a lot of my California relatives came over to help him through this tough time in his life.

Regardless of the summer's challenges, I was happy to be around the cousins who had become like brothers and sisters to me growing up. My cousin Tim shared my weight issues. We made a plan and received encouragement from Tim's brother Kevin.

While my sick family member was in the hospital, Tim, Kevin, and I pushed each other to a major wave of transformation progress. We figured we should make the summer as positive as we could. This got us out on the streets, running miles and miles each week. We all kept a low-calorie diet at the time, and although it had us feeling feeble, our combined encouragement held us to a great degree of motivation.

When the summer ended, my family member eventually made it home healthy and recovered. The fellowship was also broken between Tim, Kevin, and I. Of course, we all did our best to keep things up on our own, but we soon returned to our old ways.

While having a teammate in your journey is a wonderful benefit, depending on them to propel you through it is setting yourself up for failure.

Learn to depend on your own internal flame as it will enable you to continue with your transformation regardless of the circumstances or the people around you.

Maintaining this flame also makes you a more capable teammate to someone else, when the opportunity arises.

Mandate 6: Use Motivational Wisdom

"People often say that motivation doesn't last. Well, neither does bathing—that's why we recommend it daily."

ZIG ZIGLAR

There are many awesome individuals and programs available that can deliver an emotionally charged jolt to your day, and I have listened, watched, and read them to great benefit.

Much of their wisdom is timeless, and by listening throughout your life you'll find new meaning in their words as time goes on. Here are my favorite personalities who have many of their speeches and books available online (some for free too!):

- Les Paul
- Timothy Ferris
- Zig Ziglar
- Arnold Schwarzenegger
- Tony Robbins
- Eric Thomas
- Lou Holtz
- Kevin Smith
- Mateusz M (YouTube channel)

Listening to these people in the background is an awesome way to start the morning or commute to work, and I especially like getting pumped for a workout with some of the shorter and more intense clips.

Don't wait until you're down in the dumps to turn to a motivational speech. Listening often, even when you're feeling good, helps amp up those moods and acts like a fuel supply drop for your willpower tank throughout the day.

> "Don't let your learning lead to knowledge; let your learning lead to action."
>
> JIM ROHN,
> AMERICAN ENTREPRENEUR, AUTHOR AND MOTIVATIONAL SPEAKER

You can't wait for someone to come and tell you how to live your life, you gotta ask how other people live their lives. Become a student of the great successes you look up to. Many epic individuals have books and autobiographies that breakdown their philosophies and share the paths they took to achieve their own destiny.

You can plod through life making it up along the way, stubborn people like myself are good at that. I, however, have found the paths of my heroes to teach me different things at different times. My own path has been straightened by these mentors.

Knowing the expectations your heroes have of themselves will help you realize the expectations you should have for yourself in order to get what you desire most out of life. Who speaks to you and your life? Who inspires you? Make a point to learn about as many people's lives as you can; they can all teach us something new. Grab a book today!

✐ WRITE IT DOWN

When I read a book, I always have my **transformation journal** nearby so that I can record useful information and page numbers. My father is a staunch underliner, and his technique works marvelously. On top of this, I still find that writing down key points helps me absorb and interpret the information.

True motivation

True motivation is knowing you don't need to *feel* motivated to keep progressing. Sometimes there won't be any motivational energy when you want it. It doesn't mean anything is amiss; waves of motivation come and go like our emotions. But if you've developed habits that push you towards your goals, you'll weather motivational lulls just fine.

Those who repeatedly make it through the lull do so with a purpose that keeps them looking at the big picture, something more important than trying to fit into those slim jeans. Know your purpose, and you'll see how it shapes your decisions.

I really like to think that, over the years, my life has been expanding as I contract. I focus and weed out the things that spread my thoughts thin, enabling myself to accomplish grander dreams. If you make the effort to simplify, reduce life stressors, and conserve your willpower, you'll find that your motivational resources are more plentiful.

The potency of my progress will be magnified by inviting teammates into my quest, whether they're friends who I work alongside or mentors I look up to. If I need a little boost, I'll listen to an epic motivational monologue, or take some time to read about inspiring people. When you put all of these together, motivation will emanate from you as if you were powered by Iron Man's arc reactor.

VISUALIZE YOUR PATH

Visualization has been a part of the elite's routine for a long time now. I see it discussed time and time again, whether it's in people's autobiographies, news reports about athletes, or even scientific journals.

When we visualize a situation, we have an opportunity to formulate our actions and reactions in an ideal way. This gives us an idea of the situation playing out without actually having to experience it physically.

We use visualization all the time, most often in the form of coming up with clever comebacks to arguments we've already had while lying in bed at night. Turning the tables and becoming future-thinking enables us to be prepared for tomorrow as opposed to being resentful of yesterday.

I'll go through some of the visualization techniques I've employed to strengthen my mind. In times of waning motivation, I rely on visualization to realign my thoughts with empowering imagery. In transporting myself to the mind of the max-level, badass version of myself, I'm often inspired to live it out in reality.

Visualization Tactic 1: The Ultimate Day

Habits are all about muscle memory; the more you do a thing, the more unconscious it becomes. Visualization is a great way to build muscle memory and program habits into your life.

Think about a day where you do all the *right* things. I suggest taking some time and practicing it in your head so you have a solid target to shoot towards. Imagine in intricate detail what a good day is and use the following framework as a mental template:

- You wake up. How do you feel? Do you get out of bed gradually or do you spring out of bed like a pouncing lion?
- What's your ideal morning routine?
- What's your workday/school day/day off look like? How do you interact with the people around you?
- With what attitude do you approach the tasks of the day? Are you patient with small setbacks?
- What are you drinking, eating, snacking on?
- Do you take any breaks or walks?
- Do you use your commute (if you have one) to critique your performance, relax, or listen to audiobooks?
- What do you do during your leisure time? Exercise? Read? Write? Meditate?
- What's dinner like? Are you cooking?
- How do you prepare for sleep? What's your bedtime routine?
- What do you think about while you lie in bed before falling asleep?

Visualization Tactic 2: The Better You

From time to time I'm in situations where I make choices
I later regret. I might have ordered a big plate of nachos
when I was out with a certain group of friends or skipped
the gym and vegged out in front of the television. When I
have a small setback, I like to imagine the scene again in my
own mental theater.

Imagine making better choices instead. Get yourself into
a place where you'll be able to think in peace and play the
best version of the situation in your mind. Prepare yourself
so that when you encounter the situation again, you'll have
practiced how to better handle it.

Visualization Tactic 3: The Inner Superhero

Sometimes I lack the energy to do much. At times that I've
planned to get to the gym or be active but end up feeling
low energy, there's a visualization tactic that I commonly
use. I call this the inner superhero, and this guy is ready to
rock 24/7.

Here's what you do: turn on a good tune and imagine
yourself preparing. Imagine yourself springing off the couch,
and heading to your destination with determined focus. I
imagine myself the hero of my own movie, there to conduct
a training montage.

It's a very powerful tool that I often use. For whatever
activity you enjoy, see yourself confidently walking to the
starting position, executing movements swiftly and effi-
ciently, having the endurance to keep the pace, and finish-
ing with poise.

Many athletes use this method. The vast majority of Olympians use imagery to practice their movements and courses in the most ideal way. Even a personal hero of mine practices this kind of visualization.

> "When I was very young I visualized myself being and having what it was I wanted. Mentally I never had any doubts about it. The mind is really so incredible. Before I won my first Mr. Universe title, I walked around the tournament like I owned it. The title was already mine. I had won it so many times in my mind that there was no doubt I would win it. Then when I moved on to the movies, the same thing. I visualized myself being a famous actor and earning big money. I could feel and taste success. I just knew it would all happen."
>
> ARNOLD SCHWARZENEGGER

Visualization Tactic 4: Snapping Out of it

Emily Cook, an Olympic freestyle skier, used an interesting visualization technique whenever she noticed that a negative thought entered her mind. Realizing that her mind was becoming lost in fear of a performance or a negative score, she would immediately imagine a balloon popping. She said, "That sound and that immediate switch would kind of snap me out of it. The last couple years, I've definitely gotten to a point where, when I'm on the hill, it's very quick for me to switch from a negative thought to a positive one."[42]

When you become distracted by a negative thought or are stricken with a lack of motivation, you can look to your inner superhero. Imagine this person telling you to get up, move your butt, and stop doing whatever it is that's preventing you from reaching your goals. Similar to Emily Cook's technique, you might even imagine this person smacking you on the back of your noggin!

Visualization Tactic 5: Meditation

"Everyone dreams of the perfect vacation, in the country, by the sea, or in the mountains. You too long to get away and find that idyllic spot, yet how foolish...when at any time you are capable of finding that perfect vacation in yourself. Nowhere is there a more idyllic spot, a vacation home more private and peaceful, than in one's own mind, especially when it is furnished in such a way that the merest inward glance induces ease[...]Take this vacation as often as you like, and so charge your spirit."

MARCUS AURELIUS, ROMAN EMPEROR

Meditation is a technique that many different societies and individuals have used, most of which are outspoken in their approval and its ability to calm the mind. The practice has also been the focus of many scientific studies showing some remarkable benefits.

What we know today is that meditation:

- Improves tolerance of stress.
- Strengthens the immune system.
- Reduces blood pressure.
- Improves sleep.
- Improves attitude and outlook.
- Helps with addiction.[43]

These are only a few of the highlights. What we can take away from this research is that meditation shouldn't be overlooked. Long ago, I created a habit of a daily ten-minute meditation session where I clear my head and focus on my breathing. With just a few minutes a day, I feel that I'm more mellow, nicer, and less affected by the stresses of the day-to-day.

👍 TIP

Try this simple exercise: Start small, maybe just five minutes total, and sit in a relaxed, quiet environment. Set a timer and begin breathing steadily, focusing on those breaths. Try to keep your focus, and if you wander down a random thought path (which happens a lot), gently return to your breathing. Maintaining focus will feel almost impossible at first, but after a number of tries, it gets easier. Don't get frustrated with yourself if you find it challenging. When you're ready, extend your time to whatever length you desire.

ENVIRONMENT OF SUCCESS

> "The behavior of human beings is created by the environment. If genes predispose a certain behavior but the environment doesn't support it, then the behavior won't manifest, so in this case, genes aren't important."
>
>

The debate on nature versus nurture is out. It has been shown time and again that we are highly influenced by our surroundings. This isn't only the case during your malleable youth either, it's actually a fluid and continually evolving thing. Old or young, if you craft an environment that builds you up, you will change.

One of the pivotal points in my own transformation was related to the environment I stumbled into. It accounted for a large amount of the wind that filled my sails and propelled me to progress.

I had a significant career change in 2007 and ended up moving across the country to strike out on my own. Until then, I had been living with family when I was in town and in hotels when I was traveling for work. My home was constantly shifting and I never had a clean slate long enough to know what to do with it.

That's what this section is about: creating the kind of environment that supports your progress rather than inhibits it. While there are many influential factors on the road to transformation, you'll behandicapped overall by a poor home setting.

Charles Duhigg, author of *The Power of Habit*, discussed an interesting concept in his book called the vacation paradox. He mentions that "changing a habit on a vacation is one of the proven, most—successful ways to do it. If you want to quit smoking, you should stop smoking while you're on vacation, because all your old cues and all your old rewards aren't there anymore. So you have this ability to form a new pattern and hopefully be able to carry it over into your life."

Think about this for a minute. Have you ever noticed this happening even in a subtle way when you go on vacation? Personally, I've found that although I'm typically a night owl, when I'm on vacation, I immediately become a morning person. When I return home, this usually lasts for several days and then, after one late-night video-gaming session or Netflix series, I revert back to my old ways.

It's really surprising how variable our behavior can be, given new surroundings, and this is the clue which led me to understand one of the pillars to my own transformational success. I moved into my own apartment and learned how to use the situation as a hard reset.

The Home Environment

Home is where a lot of us spend the majority of our time away from work. It's nice to have it as comfortable as possible. We like to build up a level of luxury, and it's pretty common to attach our status to it.

But something became obvious to me only after I left the comfort I had been accustomed to at my parent's house. Comfort was a problem, a big, fluffy problem! Comfort kept me glued to the tube, comfort was keeping me only half-conscious on the couch thumbing through Facebook, and comfort made it nearly impossible for me to face these issues because I turned to it after making the statement, "I'll figure it out tomorrow."

> "Most of the luxuries, and many of the so-called comforts of life, are not only not indispensable, but positive hindrances to the elevation of mankind. With respect to luxuries and comforts, the wisest have ever lived a more simple and meagre life than the poor."
>
> HENRY DAVID THOREAU, "WALDEN"

If I had a rough day at work, my favorite thing to do was grabbing take-out from either In-N-Out Burger, Filiberto's Mexican food, or Little Caesars Pizza. Then, I would watch the tube until the pain of a gastrointestinal disturbance overshadowed the pain of my crappy job. Since all the blood in my head was whisked away to help digest food, I was in a delightful fog. For some reason, I never had enough time, even though I wasn't up to much...

When I moved, my new home was really lame by the standards I was accustomed to up to that point. It did have a television, a crappy twenty-one-incher with only local channels. At the time, I was saddened by the lack of entertainment I could access at home, but since I was broke, I couldn't afford the cable package.

I also had no access to a gaming computer anymore, as it stayed with its owner, my dad, back home. I had a clunky computer barely capable of running the graphic design software I needed for my new job. This lack of stimulus pushed me away from home and removed many of the triggers that promoted my deeply rooted bad habits.

When I visit the homes of friends and family who continue to struggle with weight, I see an environment that coaxes them into the cushions. They usually feel that, since they work as hard as they do, luxury is earned. They're resistant to giving up any of it.

You owe it to yourself to lead a life of your choosing, in a manner of opulence you feel you deserve. Nevertheless, be cautious about the evolution of your relationship with modern extravagance. The stronger you've adapted yourself to some of these advancements, the greater a challenge it will be for you to push towards a healthy and active lifestyle.

Beyond living simply, there are six rules I've adopted to help adapt my environment towards my new lifestyle.

Rule 1: Keep Your Home Clean

"I had visited Franco [Arnold's training partner and friend] many times at his room in Munich. He always kept the place extremely clean. So I knew he'd be a great roommate, and that's how it worked out. Our place was immaculate. We vacuumed regularly: the dishes were always done, with nothing piling up; and the bed was always made, military style. We were both into the discipline of getting up in the morning and straightening up before you leave the house. The more you do it, the more automatic it becomes, and the less effort it takes. Our apartment was always way cleaner than anyone else's I went to, men or women."

ARNOLD SCHWARZENEGGER

You can tell from watching shows about hoarders that people who have real clutter issues are truly consumed by it. It becomes their identity, and it weighs them down in such a procrastination slump that one messy room, which could be cleaned up in hours, eventually turns into a house full of crap. You and I may not be like this, but clutter carries with it, at every level, some tinge of stress.

We discussed how important it is to conserve your willpower energy so you can use it for what's really challenging, like new habits. Here's a good way to help loosen that button at the top of your collar: keep your place clean.

Studies conducted by UCLA and Princeton confirm that there's a universal stress response to clutter.[44] Another study was conducted at Indiana University that looked at health and how it related to the characteristics of the neigh-borhood they observed. They found that the cleanliness of a home is associated with increased physical activity and improved cardiovascular health.[45] More and more of these studies come out every year and they echo the same results.

Here are a few pointers that have done wonders to keep my life less cluttered:

- Break things down into the necessities. My mother, bless her, has a different dinner plate set for most major holidays. She has cupboards full of this stuff! If she wasn't so overwhelmed by the immensity of her collection I'd be more supportive, but the stress she feels decorating for each holiday is uncomfortable to be around...

- Spend five to ten minutes every day tidying up. My place is small, and it only takes a few minutes to keep the home in order.

- If I don't intend on using something again soon, and it's not all that expensive, I just give it away. When the need arises again, I'll buy a new one. In fact, I always have a 'donation' box slowly accumulating in the spare room. Same with a 'I don't wear this much anymore' box in the closet. When it fills up, adios!

- I'm harsh with what I'm nostalgic about. In the past, I kept all manner of mementos, but I've learned through having to clean out endless boxes of childhood junk that photographs (preferably digital) are much better to remember things by. I'm still trying to figure out how to part with my four-foot statue of Super Mario though...

- Don't postpone a clutter issue, take care of it today. Waiting till the morning might exhaust valuable willpower energy early on. I'm looking at you dishes in the sink and mail stacked on the desk

- Get rid of that junk drawer. A mess that's hidden is still there...Everything must have a place, and instead of putting things down, put them away.

By following these few simple rules, my place doesn't stress me out. When I come home, I breathe a sigh of relief and can quickly switch gears to more important tasks.

Rule 2: See the Possibilities

Since we spend so much time at home, it needs to encourage us! My home is filled with reminders of the possibilities before me. Immersing myself in this positive energy elevates my mood and keeps my eyes on the prize.

When I'm reminded of an exciting goal, or happy memory, it's as if someone is cheering me on, even if it's just my subconscious that recognizes it.

How do you get these good vibes from your home environment? It starts with a whiteboard. The whiteboard is a way for you to communicate aspirations to yourself everyday. I have mine across from my bed so that when I get up in the morning I see it straight away. I see it a few more times during the day and when I get ready for bed, I pass by it once more. Keep the whiteboard in a highly visible spot so you see it often. Eventually, your aspirations will become tattooed to your subconscious.

Here's what I like to have on my whiteboard:

- My short-term and long-term goals.
- My Habit Re-action plans, or X-Effect sheets. (if kept outside your transformation journal)
- Inspiring quotes by people I look up to.
- My travel plans for the year, organized month-to-month.
- My life purpose statement.
- Whatever else!

Furthermore, decorate your walls with photographs of your travels as a constant reminder of how much fun it is to be outside! I adore reminiscing about all the gorgeous hikes I've been on and destinations I've traveled to. Instead of sitting around wondering when the next *Half-Life* video game or season of your favorite show will come out, you'll see your own inspiring imagery, you'll be thinking about planning that next adventure...or at least going outside for a walk.

Rule 3: Stop the Screen-Binging

In today's world, screens dominate our lives. We wake up and check our phones, then head to the living room and turn on the news while getting ready for work. While we're at work, a lot of us make a living tapping away at a keyboard while looking at a computer screen, then spend our lunches scrolling through our phones. When we get home, we have to catch up on our favorite show, then back to the phone while we lay in bed waiting for the sleeping pill to kick in.

Long ago, I was basically living a life connected to the internet, like a low-bandwidth tether to the *Matrix*. If my brain wasn't absorbing some form of electronic media, I felt anxious. Have you ever felt like there's a constant need inside you to be entertained? Nowadays, if you're not *doing something* while at the coffee shop, you look insane. Like, why is that guy blankly staring off into the void, is he plotting his next murder?

With this new world, there's no reason to argue against technology, because it's here to stay. Developing a healthy relationship with our screened friends is the next best thing to throwing them all in the bin. Learning to find this balance has helped me from going totally anti-technology while still keeping myself healthy. But, truth be told, for lots of folks, technology has invited a lot of trouble.

In 1995, the island of Fiji was introduced to television. For the first time in their history, they had all of the infrastructure required to support the electricity and the necessary reception equipment.

Up until that point, the typical Fijians weren't so preoccupied with thinness as our western culture idealized. In fact, given that their culture was much more food-centric, women actually worried about *not* having an appetite, since it was a sign of ill health. A Harvard psychologist by the name of Ann Becker visited the island and was fascinated with its foodie culture, stating, "Family and social life really revolve around food....It's all about food, all the time ."[46]

She observed in 1998, after Fiji had a few years of exposure to television programming, that the number of incidents of eating disorders went from practically none to 11.3% among adolescent women. Revisiting the problem in a 2007 survey found that almost half of school-aged women who were questioned had reported purging behaviors after a meal within the last month.[46]

It might be hard to realize the effects of mass media. However, if you look at the results of its influence on more isolated locations like this one, the problems are obvious. The connections between access to media and mental health issues and disordered eating are clear.

Advertising is so hypocritical; you could potentially have a McDonald's ad selling a twenty-piece chicken Mcnugget meal followed by a cologne ad with anorexic fashion models. What do you want from us?! Oh yeah, our cash.

Furthermore, statistics show that if you watch over three hours of TV daily, which isn't hard to do, early mortality rates nearly double.[47] That's kinda scary, because I know I am way up there. Hell, I often clock three hours a day behind the screen of my laptop just writing this dang book!

Time to go for a walk. Be right back...

Part of the problem is the sedentary nature of zoning out for extended periods. But wait, there's more! Advertisers are not only feeding you marketing scientifically designed to wear away at your willpower with greasy deliciousness and photoshopped waistlines, but then we have the news channels showcasing their latest doom and gloom porn, as well as reality television instilling the lustrous virtues of back-stabbing and competitive rage.

In the home environment, technology has to take a back seat if we're going to have any willpower left to focus on other important tasks. So here's the game plan:

1. If you can, keep your phone on silent mode. Newer phones can have a feature allowing only selected individuals to actually have a ringtone, while the rest are silenced.

2. If you need to conserve your willpower fuel for the morning, try staying away from screens altogether until you've achieved your intended goal, or completed a solid morning routine.

3. For the love of sleep hygiene turn off the screen before you gear up for bed. At the very least, get that blue light filter on to give your eyes a break.

4. It's ok to turn on the tube, but try to keep your entertainment time down (less than three hours a day), and mute the advertisements or upgrade to the streaming service without them if you can afford it. (Netflix saved it's average user from 9.1 days of commercials in 2019!) [48]

5. If you have to sit for extended periods of time, especially for those who work on computers, get up at least a few times per hour.

6. Fight the urge to be constantly entertained. If there's a lull during the day, the default shouldn't be to binge on Reddit. Maybe appreciate the fluffiness of a cloud,

a pretty sunset, or that suspicious bird eyeballing your bag of chips. I'm starting to sound like a hippy now...

7. When you do screen-binge, use it as an opportunity to learn more about a hobby of interest, such as nutrition or fitness, and watch something motivating.

8. I don't let any unimportant phone apps have push notifications, they're annoying little attention robbers.

9. While I'm supposed to be spending quality time with my fellow humans, I don't pull out my phone unless I need to Google something to prove somebody wrong.

Furthermore, let's flesh out the list of negative noise sources. Keep yourself from indulging in them as best you can.

- Some major news outlets (Staying informed is great but some networks focus heavily on the negatives).
- Health "gurus" selling crap you don't need.
- Toxic Facebook feeds.
- Instagram influencers who photoshop false perfection.
- Trashy reality television.
- Gossip columns.

Be cautious about the effects and feelings mass media leaves you with. We watch the Kardashians and giggle at their misadventures. We see police chases and hope for a wreck. It's not the healthiest pastime. In today's age, we can be more selective about what we choose to fill our free time with. You'll find more peace in the hole that mass media leaves if you cut it out.

Rule 4: Keep the Junk Food Away

I quickly discovered that when I made bad habits inconvenient, I could avoid them with ease (big brain stuff right there). You must do your best to keep your home free from all the devious treats that keep it hard to stay on track.

I've gone through various stages of dieting, and one habit I adopted early on was to completely eliminate those unhealthy snack items that I once kept at home, such as candy, chips, cereal, and other junk food. If I did give myself a "blow-it" meal, I had my feast at a restaurant. Emotional eating is a significant hurdle to overcome early on, and keeping risky foods far away is paramount.

> Here's a painful (but necessary) activity. Go through your cabinets and get rid of all the things you binge on when your willpower buckles. If your significant other agrees (after you've asked them nicely to help you in your grand quest for health), get rid of their junk food too. If they won't part with the goods without a fight, place it all in a separate box or an off-limits cupboard (install a padlock if you feel you need to, I'm serious). If you like to entertain, buy a new bag of pretzels when the time comes, and give it away at the end of the night.

I could spend a day listing all the things that shouldn't be in your home that might coax you into making poor choices. I task you with making an honest list yourself. Early on I even had to rid myself of flour and sugar because there were times when I would lose all sense and bake a pile of sugar cookies for myself.

Conversely, keep healthy snacks in a really convenient, visible place. I always try to keep fruit on the counter, yogurt in the fridge, or nuts in the cupboard. When you're really craving something dastardly that would blow your plan, this is the exact thought process that should go through your head if you're on the right path:

> *You look in the cupboards, you open the fridge, you look in the cupboards again, and you look in the freezer, then you say, "Hmm, crap…" Then you think, "Maybe I should order a pizza." You confidently nope out of that idea. Then you look in the fridge again, and you stand there frustrated for about twenty seconds with your hand on your chin, possibly tapping your toes. You consider stealing from your significant other's junk food drawer, but remind yourself that it's* **off-limits.** *Finally, you grab an apple and make a cup of tea, feeling proud of yourself and thankful you didn't blow-it.*

Rule 5: Home is a Launchpad

In 2009, James Cameron released *Avatar*, a movie he'd been working on for years, and it was received with wild acclaim. I recall seeing the movie in IMAX 3D several times. It was a fun, engaging experience. Throughout the movie, I was immersed in a world so full of beauty and wonder that I recall walking out of the theater unexpectedly saddened. I remember wishing I could live in a world like that.

Many people felt the same, and the term *"Avatar* blues" was coined.[49] The sadness stemmed from people who longed to be in the beautiful jungle paradise Cameron had envisioned, yet their dreams were only realized when they closed their eyes.

At one time, I could contentedly chill at home without stepping out the door as long as there were Hot Pockets and Mountain Dew hanging around. I might have thought home had all the things I needed for happiness, but I had it wrong. Our bodies communicate another need—sunlight!

Sunlight is how our body synthesizes vitamin D, and lots of us are woefully depleted. It's said that a quarter of our population is, at some level, deficient in vitamin D, and that's quite a big deal given its link to depression, obesity, and cancer.[50] What's the prescription? The great outdoors!

These days I vaguely remember the beauty of *Avatar*'s Pandora; it doesn't captivate me like it once did. I chuckle now thinking about my own *Avatar* blues, and find it a bummer that this was such a widespread situation. We haven't given our own gorgeous planet enough attention.

There's a big, beautiful world out there. Sitting home on your luxury leather couch and viewing it through David Attenborough's documentaries isn't the way to experience it.

"There"s one life to live,
And too much outdoors for me to be sittin' in the crib."

MAIN SOURCE, "TIME"

One way I've influenced myself to get out and see more is by thinking of home as a launchpad. Instead of building luxury, I have what I need and keep it simple. Instead of investing in couches you sink into and huge entertainment centers, things that would make me want to veg out, I invest in stuff that helps me hike, camp, and play outside. My mental health has truly benefited from this less needy home environment, so too can yours.

The Ultimate Habitat

There's more clarity of mind in an orderly home environment that supports healthy habits. You'll have less battles with yourself about what to eat and feel more encouraged to get outside or go to the gym. When you see your goals first thing in the morning, you'll start your day on track with this reminder of your intention. Life will get busy though, and sometimes you'll be chilling out, feeling like you're low on fuel. Good thing the addictive junk foods are harder to access. These times are excellent chances to test your screen-binging habits. At the very least, we can learn about something interesting or helpful. If there's no intellectual energy to be found, we can try to keep the TV time under three hours. A while before bed, we should log off and give our eyes a rest so we can start the new day fresh. Lastly, leave your worries at home, venture forth outside and let the sun kiss your skin as often as you're able. Don't forget the sunblock.

THE POSITIVE MINDSET

> "You will truly be cheerful in life the day that you realize that no matter what is happening around you, being anything other than cheerful will not make it any better."
>
> TONY ROBBINS,
> AMERICAN BUSINESSMAN, AUTHOR, AND PHILANTHROPIST

There's no doubt that for those of us who struggle with weight, positive thinking will be an issue. But a passive issue it is not. Beyond the foundational elements of the transformation, like goal setting, diet, and exercise, your perspective, positive or not, will cast its light over it all. The right mindset is pivotal in becoming your better self. Positive thinking will:

- Keep your willpower energy high so that you can become a better and more effective decision maker.
- Allow belief that there is a light at the end of the tunnel if you're going through hell.
- Help you to be likeable. Others will notice, and some will be mentors whose help you'll appreciate.
- Spread good vibes and inspire others. Some will see you as a mentor.
- Find solutions, whereas negativity is self-fulfilling.

For quite a while, negativism was at the root of my problems. The barometer for my success in life was only measuring the external—the money I didn't have in my bank account, the people who I was lagging behind, and the fat guy I saw in the mirror. I thought in terms of who I wasn't.

By only looking at these factors, you'll never be able to make peace with who you are at each step along your own journey. The first concept I want to emphasize in terms of having a positive mindset is that we all have value, no matter where we are in relation to our dreams.

You Have Value

You have value, fat or skinny, rich or poor. You're not a substandard human because of who you are; it's only your own thoughts that will ever make that seem true. Being thin does not make you a better human, and might not even make you healthier depending on how you get there.

When I was younger, I had a shortsighted view of myself in the mirror. I was fat, sick, down on myself, and felt pretty worthless sometimes. I may have been fat and sick, but I wouldn't always be so. I saw my stunted growth as a reason to think less of myself. But I didn't give myself credit for trying again and again, or for developing the good virtues I'm proud of today. Transforming yourself is a lifelong process! Are you as much of a hardass on yourself as I was?

I wrote this book not only to help others, but as a way to have a conversation with the younger version of myself. The first thing I'd do is let younger me know that the path literally can not be a straight line. You have to ping-pong all over the place for a while. It's still freakin' like that! Real life has taught me that smooth-sailing success is a concept that Hollywood came up with.

We all have value, right now, so don't wait until you look a certain way in the mirror for you to start believing in your own. If you've messed up and feel like you're right back at the starting line, remember that you still gained some experience along the way, even if you didn't level up. I mean, look at you right now, taking steps to better yourself. That's excellent!

This leads us to an important rule, one I learned to abide by through the highs and lows of my transformation.

Be Kind to Yourself

One of my friends, let's call him Greg, is intelligent and skilled in many ways, obvious to all but him, it would seem. Greg has some amazing qualities but is also haunted by a darkness that often boils up. He perpetually talks down to himself.

When I get the opportunity to spend time with him, I always feel like I should have a spray bottle filled with water so I can spritz him each time he gets down on himself, as if he was a misbehaving kitty cat.

I'm disheartened by the frequency with which he starts sentences with phrases like "I was such an idiot for...," and "I always find a way of screwing things up." But the truth is, at one point, I was just as guilty of the same mental habits as he is now.

Now that you understand the perception he has of himself, what do you think his perception of society is? If you guessed that he feels people are cruel and life is inherently unfair, you're correct.

Interestingly enough, this relationship between internal and external perceptions has been studied. A meta-analysis of several correlating studies show that those who perceive themselves to be less attractive also believed in a greater social inequality.[51]

Want to make the world a better place? You can start by boosting your opinion of yourself.

The moment you give in to thoughts that you are undeserving, a loser, or ugly, they transfer their power to your actions, sometimes in the most subtle ways. You act the way a loser would act; you have sour thoughts of your lot in life because you feel, deep down, that this is how you should behave.

> "Watch your thoughts for they become words.
> Watch your words for they become actions.
> Watch your actions for they become habits.
> Watch your habits for they become your character.
> And watch your character for it becomes your destiny."
>
> MARGARET THATCHER,
> FORMER PRIME MINISTER OF THE UNITED KINGDOM

If you think experiencing success is a challenge or you think losing a bunch of weight is a struggle, try waking up every day trapped in a mental and physical prison that can literally tint the world in a negative light. If you don't choose to think well of yourself, then you're in this prison, too. Break out!

From now on, even if you find it hard, you will talk yourself up with your voice and your thoughts. You must fight the tendency to down-talk at all costs. **You are a work in progress at the worst, nothing less.**

> 👍 TIP
>
> If bringing awareness to the white noise of your mind makes you realize that you down-talk quite often, you might wear a rubber band around your wrist, snapping it each time you notice the problem. Recall our visualization tactic (tactic number four) of the popping balloon, as well, or the inner mentor. They can be a quick jolt of lightning to the mind and will help you bring about better thoughts.

The Highway

How do we create a self-generating system for better thoughts? By taking them on one by one.

Think of your mind as a small city with a large system of roads. Your mind is ceaselessly sending construction crews to either maintain or improve some of the roads, and withdrawing maintenance crews from roadways that no longer serve a purpose. Thoughts are the vehicles that travel these roadways, and depending on your disposition and other factors, traffic will travel to and fro.

The system isn't perfect, though. Sometimes the roadways that lead to negativity become reinforced so much that your

GPS software tells you to go that way even though there may be a healthier route. Your GPS will favor familiarity over better options. Unfortunately, for a lot of us, negative routes are superhighways with eight lanes and rubberized asphalt.

If your brain sees all the traffic heading a certain way, it will send the highway improvement crew to that road. Sometimes, this is to your detriment! **These negativity roadways, while having eight lanes and being smooth as glass to drive on, have a toll booth. Each time you travel it, you lose something.** When you let a negative thought enter, you pay a price to travel that road, and the toll will eat away at you bit by bit. Eventually, the drain on your psychological wallet becomes staggering.

If you want to maintain your sanity and give yourself the best opportunity possible to live a good life, you must fight the urge to drive that toll road no matter how convenient it may seem.

The roads you let your thoughts travel on are the roads that get improved. You want positivity to be the superhighway with the eight lanes and rubberized asphalt, not the negativity one with the toll booth. To do this, you must take that overgrown dirt trail that leads up the mountain hill. This road may not have gotten much traffic lately, but after driving on it a dozen times, your tires will smooth out the bumps. Eventually, if you work at it hard enough, it will become a more efficient method of travel. Not only will the city recognize that this road gets all the traffic and forget about maintaining that other road, but you'll actually gain something at the end of it as well.

For me, that negative road still exists, but it's got cracks, some potholes even, and when I drive down it these days I'm reminded of why I started taking the other road, and quickly get off at the nearest exit.

You need to stop giving your brain a reason to improve the negativity highway. To do that, you must stop traveling down it. It wasn't until I realized this simple fact that I started to monitor the kinds of thoughts I let pass through my mind.

Now that you have a basic understanding about the principles of how the positive mindset works, let's get ourselves on a better foundation.

Was it Bad Luck to Have Become Unhealthy?

A big step in my quest for positivity was deciding that maybe becoming fat and sick wasn't a purely negative event. For a time, I couldn't fathom what could possibly be good about all those troubled years.

I'd like to share an old Zen story I had the pleasure of hearing once:

"This farmer had only one horse, and one day the horse ran away. The neighbors came to console him over his terrible loss. The farmer said, "What makes you think it is so terrible?"

A month later, the horse came home, this time bringing with her two beautiful wild horses. The neighbors became excited at the farmer's good fortune. Such lovely strong horses! The farmer said, "What makes you think this is good fortune?"

The farmer's son was thrown from one of the wild horses and broke his leg. All the neighbors were very distressed. Such bad luck! The farmer said, "What makes you think it is bad?"

A war came, and every able-bodied man was conscripted and sent into battle. Only the farmer's son, because he had a broken leg, remained. The neighbors congratulated the farmer. "What makes you think this is good?" said the farmer."[52]

This illustrates the incredibly important idea about the inability to see what the future holds. It's easy to perceive something as either good or bad in the moment. However, **We can only connect the dots looking back, and perhaps, something we deem as terrible in the moment could, in fact, be something that caused us to grow and learn in unexpected ways.**

Think about examples in your own life. Some of the roughest chapters of my life left, in their wake, a much stronger me. This is completely true for my own transformation, and I'm certain you will share the same sentiment.

To this end, you don't have to feel so bummed about how things are. I feel lucky to have learned how to rise above my weight problem. The lessons I learned will always stay with me and are responsible for all of the successes I'm proud of now.

Since we don't know our future, we should believe that our efforts *will* bring us good things, even if it's taking time.

With a positive mindset, you can make any tragedy in your own life a great triumph.

Rationalizing

It can be unconscious to shift the weight of responsibility off our shoulders and onto other people or the current situation. Hell, you might even have a good point in blaming something that seems to be sabotaging your struggle for a better self! But that's besides the point, because our actions are always the result of our decisions. Here are a few examples of some common blaming techniques we often use:

- This is just how my parents raised me.
- If my significant other would stop bringing home junk food I could get on the right track.
- How can I ever make progress if the world is designed to keep me fat!

Practice accepting responsibility for the decisions you make, regardless of extenuating circumstances. This extends to any grief you might lend to your upbringing.

Arnold Schwarzenegger said, "Don't blame your parents. They've done their best for you, and if they've left you with problems, those problems are now yours to solve."[53] You don't get to choose how you were brought into this world. Your parents, good or bad, are yours to love, or at the very least, learn from. Glean the lessons from the environment they raised you in.

I love my parents, and although the direction my youth took was, in some manner, out of my control, there's no sense in being resentful about it. My parents did their best in a complex world, and I am grateful for every opportunity I had because of them.

Whatever your past can teach you, extract the positives and the lessons, and leave the rest to the wind. Dwelling on injustices of days past only contributes to a bitter outlook going forward. These thoughts have no place in your life. In the end, your actions are your responsibility, and so is your future. Focus on that.

The Devastating Path of Self-pity

"It's not who you are that holds you back, it's who you think you're not."

DENIS WAITLEY, AMERICAN MOTIVATIONAL SPEAKER

As a Joe Schmoe in the sea of society, it's sometimes hard to see our own unique gifts. We're all built differently and will excel at different things. From a young age, we're treated more as a group and less as individuals, and this can make us feel insecure because of natural differences between us.

Given all these differences, some people can naturally develop shame about their lot. It's often the result of comparing ourselves to others. A great many things lay out of your control, and some will get into the fast lane and easily sail past with seemingly little effort.

Should chance cause another kid to be born into a wealthy family, would it be rational to think of yourself as a loser because you're poor? Of course not! It doesn't make any sense to think that way.

For some, it takes a lot of trial and error to eventually find their own way. I think that's the story for a lot of us dealing with weight issues; we're just in the process of finding our way to health.

When I dropped out of college, a lot of my friends seemed like they were cruising through their lives like everything was easy. They were looking healthy, getting college degrees, getting married, having babies, buying houses, etc...I dropped out of college, was morbidly obese, single, and was working a dead-end job.

I really gave into self pity. I looked at where all my friends were, and saw myself as a bigtime loser. I spent so much time feeling sorry for myself, when it might have been more self-compassionate to consider it my own learning process. This is called self pity, and it will suck all the wind from your sails.

"Certainly the most destructive vice if you like, that a person can have. More than pride, which is supposedly the number one of the cardinal sins - is self-pity. Self pity is the worst possible emotion anyone can have. And the most destructive... Self pity will destroy relationships, it'll destroy anything that's good, it will fulfill all the prophecies it makes and leave only itself. And it's so simple to imagine that one is hard done by, and that things are unfair, and that one is underappreciated, and that if only one had had a chance at this, only one had had a chance at that, things would have gone better, you would be happier if only this, that one is unlucky. All those things. And some of them may well even be true. But, to pity oneself as a result of them is to do oneself an enormous disservice."

STEPHEN FRY, ENGLISH COMEDIAN, WRITER, AND ACTOR

Self-pity hobbles empowerment, cancels solution-oriented thinking, and everything you need to get back on your feet. It's just a brick wall.

Instead of building a wall, we've got to rise above self-pity. Truth is, you're far from powerless. Ask yourself if you spend any ounce of your energy thinking these thoughts:

- I always get the short end of the stick.
- I'm underappreciated.
- If only I'd had a chance, things might be different.
- I don't deserve this. What have I done to deserve this?
- I'm not good enough, smart enough, etc. No wonder things aren't working out.
- So-and-so has it so much better. Why can't I be lucky like him/her?

The world isn't designed to be fair, so it's up to us to get to where we want to be from wherever we are. **Don't dwell on misfortune any longer than it takes to understand how to get past it and rise above.** In the words of Marcus Aurelius, "It's up to you!"

Eventually, you will reach a point where you feel good about yourself. These lessons learned in the trenches will be ingrained into your mind so deeply that you'll never forget them.

Also, instead of looking at others with jealousy, you'll see them as people that deserve all the good things that life has to offer. Getting to that point takes time, and if you're already there, then badass. By digging deep and discovering what inspires you, and then pursuing those things, you'll create a strong sense of worthiness. Everything we've talked about up to this point will help with that.

Until you believe it in your heart, accept that you are worthy. You are worthy of living a good life, of being happy, healthy, and having success. The learning curve for some is steep, as it was for me, but we will get there together. The more effort you place on bettering yourself, the more you'll undoubtedly agree.

THE FAST LANE

Achieving our goals gives us one important thing, the understanding that we have power, that we aren't slaves to the forces around us. It gives us a sense of freedom. The victory of each individual milepost is nice for a while, but the lasting effects are the knowledge that we're on the right path.

You aren't helpless. You are the master of your own destiny, whatever that means to you. There are many paths and it's up to you which one you'll take. Once you believe in yourself, things change. The challenge turns into a game, problems give way to solutions, and the world becomes a big playground.

> *"Once a small win has been accomplished, forces are set in motion that favor another small win."[1]*

Eventually, you get to a point where your small victories blur together. You keep accomplishing your short-term goals and the long-term goal now seems like something more than a fanciful wish. It isn't a dream, and that's the truth. People tend to magnify the difficulty, but in the end it's baby steps that bring us to a better life; bit by bit, large goals are simply a collection of obtainable, bite-sized pieces. Welcome to the fast lane! Recognize your success and feed off of the feeling of accomplishing these challenges.

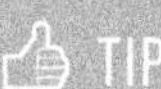

👍 TIP

What are some cool things to do as the weight comes off?

- Since you now fit into smaller clothes, reward your weight loss milestones with a new outfit.
- List some items you want but which aren't necessarily needed, and place them in weight loss increments of ten to twenty pounds. When you reach certain milestones, treat yourself to a new, fun thing.
- Post a message in an online forum or bulletin board about your success and include some details. It's great to receive feedback and encouragement while inspiring others.
- One person I spoke with mentioned she has a charm bracelet and, when she reaches a certain weight loss milestone, she buys a new charm for it. How cool it would be to see those charms build up!
- Take some pictures and compare them to your original progress pictures.

- Show some more skin! As an exercise in building confidence I recommend hiking or running shirtless (guys) or with an exposed midriff (girls).

Complacency & Fat Acceptance

I applaud any level of transformation that a well-intentioned person achieves. I also think that it is very easy to become complacent with successes that feel good enough. Is good enough ok? This is a question you have to ask yourself.

I'll never suggest that obtaining the ripped look should be the goal for all, and might even go a step further in suggesting that a lot of the reason why I wanted that look was for vanity's sake. Be honest with yourself and your desires.

There's absolutely nothing wrong with having a few extra pounds, and learning to love yourself regardless of how you compare to the men and women of the magazine ads is a lifelong skill. This is not fat acceptance, this is self-compassion. Obesity, however, can and should be conquered.

"Beauty is in the eye of the beholder, but health is science."

BILL MAHER, AMERICAN COMEDIAN AND TALK SHOW HOST

If you are happy with yourself—thin, obese, tall or short—then fantastic. But let's not avoid the science that overwhelmingly rejects the "bigger is better" claim. We need to support each other's pursuits **for health**, and show love and compassion for every shape and for people in every stage of their journey.

ACCOMPLISHING THE LONG-TERM GOAL AND THE NEW LIFESTYLE

What did I find at the end of the road? Did I find everything that I was hoping I would? Not immediately, of course not. Weight loss is just another mile marker on this path—but let me tell you, making it to the long-term goal was amazing.

There will forever be stamped in my memory the night I walked into the gym and made my way to the body fat analysis machine, which I had been using to measure my progress. I knew I was close and when the machine told me that I was under 10% body fat (my original long-term goal, set YEARS before) I had something I can only describe as a moment where time stood still. The moment *was* amazing, but in truth it pales in comparison to how well my life had already changed leading up to it.

So, did I stay ripped? The short answer is no, and it might be surprising to read that (or maybe not!). In the process, I developed such a keen sense of self-worth that I didn't need my body to have *that look*. What this meant was not that I stopped exercising, or stopped eating healthy, but that I became more relaxed with my diet. I allowed a slice of pizza now and then and stopped keeping track of every calorie. I took a few years off from focusing on weightlifting, and started running and surfing more. Sometimes I would be a total homebody and play through a new videogame.

I found, after many years, that maintaining my weight in a ten-pound range of what I thought of as "being ripped" was actually surprisingly doable. This maintenance required only continuing on with my healthy lifestyle. Doesn't that sound like the right way to live? We can all get there.

For fun, I have found it quite possible to refocus my attention on getting back *the look* and have occasionally returned to it for fear it will be forever lost. It certainly is achievable again and is comforting to know that the lessons in this guide continue to ring true in different stages of my life.

What used to be so hard, like heading to the gym, going for a jog, eating vegetables and going days and weeks without a major blow-it, is a non-issue these days. I mean, don't get me wrong, I can still eat a whole pizza in one sitting, and have been known to utterly ruin my appetite because the wife decided to bake a pile of cookies. But I digress...

I find that the little successes of eating a healthy meal, doing something fun that gets my heart rate up, learning something new, pursuing new goals—all of these make life a continually enjoyable process. Victory is found in living a good, balanced, healthy life, things I wholeheartedly believe are achievable for everyone who makes it a priority.

Years and Decades, Not Days and Months

One of the hardest concepts for me to accept was that of years and decades. This is the timeline for real change, for real transformations. We've seen some superpowered people blast through six months of carnage to get down to their goal weight, and those before and after photos can be so remarkable. I applaud their drive, but I think it gives a lot of people an unrealistic expectation of themselves.

Instead, think of the timeline in years and decades. Will you be thin and healthy in a decade? A crash diet will, more than likely, not bring you to that reality since long-term transformation is found by reengineering your mind and habits.

I learned that this extended timeline is prevalent with other parts of my life, be it career success, fitness goals, or even in relationships. Developing and nurturing an important life goal isn't something that should be rushed through like you're taking shortcuts to get home during rush hour. Taking time to appreciate the nuances of the experience will add longevity to lessons learned.

So, remember that you won't always find success within days and months, even though some do. Going from 300 pounds to 180 took me almost a decade. That's a long-ass time, but since time always marches on, better late than never.

Regret

Regrets can stack up like fortress walls. It was easy to think that I had amassed insurmountable regret and that my life would be overshadowed by the unfortunate decisions I made early on in life. I'd say, "even *if* I lose the weight, stretch marks and maybe even droopy skin will haunt me forever." While I do have loose skin and stretch marks, I was otherwise completely wrong!

> "The strange thing is, everything washed up from the sea was purified."
>
> HARUKI MURAKAMI,
> "HARD-BOILED WONDERLAND AND THE END OF THE WORLD"

The ocean takes broken bottles, sharp and coarse, and grinds them into beautiful colored rocks. Likewise, regrets of my past and all those rough patches I went through have been smoothed out. So long as you don't keep throwing in more trash, it will get better.

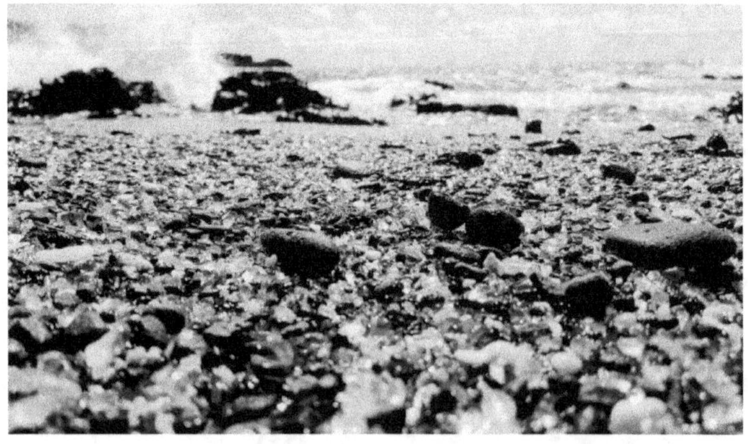

For fun, here are some pros and cons from my transformation:

PROS

- Shopping for clothes isn't *as* demoralizing as it used to be. (Generally, I'm still not a fan.)
- I'm way less picky about food, and cook tons. People tell me I'm good at it.
- I scored my dream girl, and put a ring on her!
- I'm not depressed anymore. Although, my wife says I'm moody sometimes. I think that's normal, right?
- My legs can walk really far. I'm still not great at running but I *tried* a marathon, which was a fun experience.
- My cholesterol is great, blood pressure is vastly improved (totally off medications), and I have a resting heart rate that is usually in the fifties.

CONS

- Still have stretch marks and loose skin. (But it doesn't bother me nearly as much as I thought it might!)
- Apparently, I wasn't gassy *because* my body was trying to exemplify the fat guy cliche, because I'm still gassy...
- I probably check myself out in the mirror too much.
- I *do* have binge-eating episodes. I find that the best bet for me is limiting carbs and mindful eating techniques.
- I'm still generally nervous showing skin in public situations, but I definitely do, and with much more confidence.
- Because I was so judgemental with myself, I find that I can be judgmental towards others. But I'm really working on that.

We're in this Together

You're not alone in your struggles; there are many others going through it as well as people who have already accomplished the magical journey of transforming themselves. Sometimes I think about how awesome it would be if I could have been there for my younger self. I definitely would have a lot to say.

I didn't just create these ideas out of thin air, no way. I educated myself from the blood, sweat, and tears of others. I always had guidance and people were most certainly there for me. Their lessons came from countless places in the past and present finding me. Those who have succeeded are there for you too.

I know we can't teleport ideas back in time, but it gives me comfort to imagine this book magically arriving on lil' me's lap one night. I see him sitting there frustrated, lost, and confused. He opens the book and can't put it down. I want him to be excited and I want him to have direction. I want him to start walking on the path to self-betterment the next morning, confident in knowing he is finally on the right one.

Make a pact with me right now that when you see your transformation through, you'll pass on what you've learned just as my mentors have. There are a great many lost and troubled individuals out there who need direction in their own lives. Each of us has a different story, and the path we took, our struggles, can be of help.

"Nothing, however outstanding and however helpful, will ever give me any pleasure if the knowledge is to be for my benefit alone. If wisdom were offered to me on the one condition that I should keep it shut away and not divulge it to anyone, I should reject it. There is no enjoying the possession of anything valuable unless one has someone to share it with."

And don't ever say that nobody believes in you, because I do. If you wish to contact me, please do so through my website at Blurrylife.com/contact/. Please be patient with me as I will do my best to respond.

ACKNOWLEDGEMENTS

I'm very thankful to those who've had an impact in the making of this book. In no particular order, thanks to the following:

- Sonia Jones for being a motivating instructor in the Fire Academy and good friend.
- Jason Jones for taking an out of shape kid to the Grand Canyon, that really amped up my self-confidence, sorry about Krempining you so many times.
- My darling wife Mitsy for suffering with me on our intrepid adventures.
- Beth Danowski for helping me smooth out my ideas on food and nutrition.
- My invaluable editors Courtney Meunier and Lee Allen Howard.
- Any friend who cringed their way through earlier versions of the book...
- Mom and Dad for always being there for me.
- Brian for being a good friend and encouraging people to follow a healthy path.

ABOUT THE AUTHOR

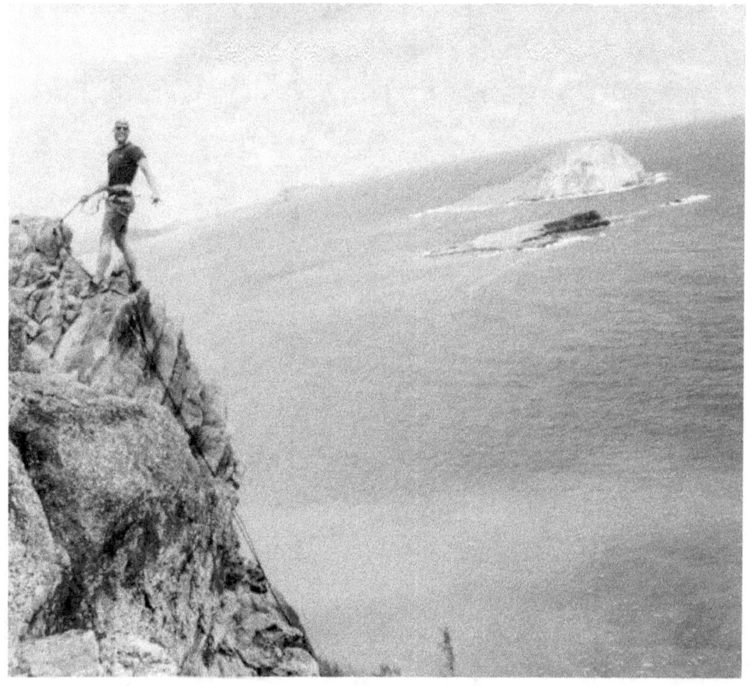

With this new body, I've discovered a new way of life. Since I left behind my old self and wrote this book, many things have changed. I've discovered a love for travel and rekindled my love for the outdoors. My wife and I live in Hawaii and take every chance to explore the world and go on cool adventures. Since Orizaba, some of the more notable adventures include summiting Kilimanjaro in 2018 and venturing to Everest Basecamp in 2019. I'm not sure what lies ahead, but I am more than stoked for the future. Check out BlurryLife.com for more.

DISCLAIMER

Before starting any new diet and exercise program, please check with your doctor and clear any exercise or diet changes before you begin. I am not a doctor or registered dietitian; I am a registered nurse with less academic background on these topics. I do not claim to cure any condition or disease.

This book shares my opinions regarding personal experience. The information and research covered in this book is cited and open to the public. I am not liable, either expressly or in an implied manner, nor claim any responsibility for any emotional or physical problems that may occur directly or indirectly from reading this book.

Children and adolescents, pregnant or breastfeeding women, and people with significant health problems such as bulimia, heart disease, kidney disease, diabetes or psychiatric disorders, should not begin any fitness or diet program without written authorization from their primary care provider.

People under treatment for other conditions or taking medications prescribed by their healthcare provider should tell their providers that they have begun a diet because, in some cases, adjustments to medications or modifications to the weight loss program may be appropriate.

RESOURCES

[1] Duhigg, Charles. *The Power of Habit: Why We Do What We Do in Life and Business* New York: Random House (2012).

[2] Warren Buffett's "2 List" Strategy: How to Maximize Your Focus and Master Your Priorities (n.d.). James Clear. Retrieved from https://jamesclear.com/buffett-focus

[3] "Keep your goals to yourself," Derek Sivers, http://www.ted.com/talks/derek_sivers_keep_your_goals_to_yourself?language=en

[4] "When Intentions go public: does social reality widen the intention-behavior gap?" Gollwitzer, P .M., Sheeran, P., Michalski, V., & Sheifert A.E. (2009). *Psychological Science*, 20(5),612-618. https://doi.org10.1111/j.1467-9280.2009.02336

[5] "Fatty foods may cause cocaine-like addiction," Sarah Klein, Health.com, http://www.cnn.com/2010/HEALTH/03/28/fatty.foods.brain/index.html

[6] "Emotional eating in overweight, normal weight, and underweight individuals." Geliebter, Allan, and Angela Aversa. *Eating Behaviors* vol. 3,4 (2003): 341-7. doi:10.1016/s1471-0153(02)00100-9

[7] Albers, S. (2009). *50 Ways to Soothe Yourself Without Food.* Oakland: New Harbinger Publications.

[8] "Mindfulness definition," https://www.psychologytoday.com/basics/mindfulness

[9] "Habit definition," http://www.merriam-webster.com/dictionary/habit

[10] "Long-term weight loss maintenance." Wing, R. R., & Phelan, S. (2005, July 1). *The American Journal of Clinical Nutrition*, 82(1), 222-225. https://doi.org/10.1093/ajcn/82.1.222S

[11] FourHourBodyPress. (2011, March 16). Richard Branson on Exercise and Productivity [Video File]. Retrieved from https://www.youtube.com/watch?v=QFjgMKwpz_k

[12] "The Ex Effect," Bombjoke http://www.reddit.com/r/getdisciplined/comments/1x99m6/im_a_piece_of_shit_no_more_games_no_more_lies_no/cf9dz72

[13] "How are habits formed: Modelling habit formation in the real world," European Journal of Social Psychology, Volume 40, Issue 6, pages 998–1009, October 2010, Phillippa Lally, Cornelia H. M. van Jaarsveld, Henry W. W. Potts and Jane Wardle

[14] "Contributions to anthropological splanchnology. I. Racial studies on the large intestine," Edward L. Miloslavich, American Journal of Physical Anthropology, Volume 8, Issue 1, pages 11–22, January/March 1925, http://onlinelibrary.wiley.com/doi/10.1002/ajpa.1330080102/abstract

[15] "Got Lactase? Understanding Evolution 2016" by The University of California Museum of Paleontology, Berkeley, and the Regents of the University of California, http://evolution.berkeley.edu/evolibrary/news/070401_lactose

[16] "Geographical variation of human gut micro-bial composition," Taichi A. Suzuki, Michael Worobey, *Biology Letters,* Published 12 February 2014. DOI: 10.1098/rsbl.2013.1037 http://rsbl.royalsociety-publishing.org/content/10/2/20131037.abstract?sid=0f89b697-8df8-4c1e-8ecf-48712010cb44

[17] Willcox, B. J., Willcox, D. C., & Suzuki, M. (2002, March 12). The Okinawa Program: How the World's Longest-Lived People Achieve Everlasting Health--And How You Can Too. New York: Random House.

[18] Fung, J. (2016, March 3). The Obesity Code: Unlocking the Secrets of Weight Loss. British Columbia, CA: Greystone Books.

[19] Pulcinella, M. (2012, August 8). "Kai Greene: A Day in the Life" Part ⅓ [Video File]. Retrieved from https://www.youtube.com/watch?v=TRGCNlk4RSo

[20] "The 90% rule for eating well and enjoying your food," Precision Nutrition, John Berardi, Ph.D., http://www.precisionnutrition.com/day-2

[21] "Effects of Dietary Fiber and Its Components on Metabolic Health." Lattimer, J. M., & Haub, M. D. (2010, December 15). *Nutrients,* 2(12), 1266-1289. https://doi.org/10.3390/nu2121266

[22] "Protein: Which is Best?" 2004 Sep; 3(3): 118–130. Jay R. Hoffman, Michael J. Falvo, *Journal of Sports Science & Medicine,* http://www.ncbi.nlm.nih.gov/pmc/articles/PMC3905294/

[23] "How can obese weight controllers minimize weight gain during the holiday season? By self-monitoring very consistently." Boutelle KN, Kirschenbaum DS, Baker RC, Mitchell ME, *Health Psychology*, 18:364-68, 1999. http://www.ncbi.nlm.nih.gov/pubmed/10431937

[24] "Phelps' Pig Secret: He's Boy Gorge," Lisi Clemente, http://nypost.com/2008/08/13/phelps-pig-secret-hes-boy-gorge/

[25] "After The Biggest Loser, Their Bodies Fought to Regain Weight," Gina Kolata, New York Times, http://www.nytimes.com/2016/05/02/health/biggest-loser-weight-loss.html

[26] "A new predictive equation for resting energy expenditure in healthy individuals". Mifflin MD, St Jeor ST, Hill LA, Scott BJ, Daugherty SA, Koh YO (1990). *American Journal of Clinical Nutrition* 51 (2): 241–7. PMID 2305711.

[27] "The myth of 1 g/lb: Optimal protein intake for bodybuilders," Menno Henselmans, http://bayesianbodybuilding.com/the-myth-of-1glb-optimal-protein-intake-for-bodybuilders/

[28] "Macronutrient content of a hypoenergy diet affects nitrogen retention and muscle function in weight lifters." Walberg JL, Leidy MK, Sturgill DJ, Hinkle DE, Ritchey SJ, Sebolt DR.

[29] "Protein requirements and muscle mass/strength changes during intensive training in novice bodybuilders." Lemon PW, Tarnopolsky MA, MacDougall JD, Atkinson SA.

[30] "Effect of Protein Intake on Strength, Body Composition and Endocrine Changes in Strength/Power Athletes," Jay R

Hoffman, corresponding author Nicholas A Ratamess, Jie Kang, Michael J Falvo, and Avery D Faigenbaum.

[31] "How much protein do I need every day?" Alex Leaf, http://examine.com/faq/how-much-protein-do-i-need-every-day/

[32] "Persistent metabolic adaptation 6 years after The Biggest Loser competition," Obesity 5/2016, Erin Fothergill, Juen Guo, Lilian Howard, Jennifer C. Kerns, Nicolas D. Knuth, Robert Brychta, Kong Y. Chen, Monica C. Skarulis, Mary Walter, Peter J. Walter and Kevin D. Hall, http://onlinelibrary.wiley.com/doi/10.1002/oby.21538/abstract

[33] Csikszentmihalyi, M. (2009, October 13). Flow: The Psychology of Optimal Experience. New York: HarperCollins.

[34] PowerfulJRE. (2018, June 19). JRE MMA Show #32 with Firas Zahabi [Video File]. Retrieved from https://www.youtube.com/watch?v=xDsoWp743gM

[35] "Play Doesn't End With Childhood: Why Adults Need Recess Too," Sami Yenigun, https://www.npr.org/sections/ed/2014/08/06/336360521/play-doesnt-end-with-childhood-why-adults-need-recess-too

[36] "The association between school-based physical activity, including physical education, and academic performance: a systematic review of the literature." Rasberry, C. N., Lee, S. M., Robin, L., Laris, B. A., Russel, L. A., Coyle, K. K., & Nihiser, A. J. (2011). *Preventative Medicine*, 52(1), 10-20. https://doi.org/10.1016/j.ypmed.2011.01.027.

[37] "The Case Against Stretching" Hutchinson, A. (2020, January 30). *Outside* Retrieved from https://www.outsideonline.com/2408467/case-against-stretching-flexibility-research

[38] "Self-determination theory and the facilitation of intrinsic motivation, social development, and well-being". Ryan, R. M.; Deci, E. L. (2000). *American Psychologist*, 55 (1): 68–78. doi:10.1037/0003-066X.55.1.68

[39] "Self-Determined Motivation as a Predictor of Burnout Among College Athletes." Holmberg, P. M., & Sheridan, D. A. (2013). *The Sport Psychologist*, 27(2), 177-187. https://doi.org/10.1123/tsp.27.2.177

[40] "The Social Readjustment Rating Scale". Holmes TH, Rahe RH (1967). *J Psychosom Res* 11 (2): 213–8. doi:10.1016/0022-3999(67)90010-4. PMID 6059863

[42] "Stanford research shows that working together boosts motivation," Clifton B. Parker http://news.stanford.edu/news/2014/september/motivation-walton-carr-091514.html

[43] "Olympians Use Imagery as Mental Training," Christopher Clarey, New York Times http://www.nytimes.com/2014/02/23/sports/olympics/olympians-use-imagery-as-mental-training.html?_r=0

[44] "Interactions of Top-Down and Bottom-Up Mechanisms in Human Visual Cortex," Stephanie McMains, Sabine Kastner; *Journal of Neuroscience* 12 January 2011, 31 (2) 587-597; DOI: 10.1523/JNEUROSCI.3766-10.2011

[45] "Tidier homes, fitter bodies?" https://newsinfo.iu.edu/webpage/normal/14627.html

[46] "Fijian girls succumb to Western dysmorphia," Anne E. Becker, http://news.harvard.edu/gazette/story/2009/03/fijian-girls-succumb-to-western-dysmorphia/

[47] "Can too much TV be deadly?" Hoai-Tran Bui, Http://www.usatoday.com/story/news/nation/2014/06/25/tv-television-early-death-premature-risk-sedentary/11366047/

[48] Toledo, R. (2020, May 15). ANALYSIS: Netflix Saved Its Average User From 9.1 Days of Commercials in 2019, Reviews.com. Retrieved from https://www.reviews.com/entertainment/streaming/netflix-hours-of-commercials-analysis/

[49] "Audiences experience 'Avatar' blues," Jo Piazza, http://www.cnn.com/2010/SHOWBIZ/Movies/01/11/avatar.movie.blues/

[50] "Vitamin D Deficiency and Depression," Dale Archer M.D., https://www.psychologytoday.com/blog/reading-between-the-headlines/201307/vitamin-d-deficiency-and-depression

[51] "Mirror, mirror on the wall, who's the fairest of them all? Thinking that one is attractive increases the tendency to support inequality," Peter Belmi, Margaret Neale, https://www.gsb.stanford.edu/sites/gsb/files/publication-pdf/Belmi%20Neale%20Mirror%20Mirror%20OBHDP.pdf

[52] Hancock, E. (1993). Editor's Note, *Johns Hopkins Magazine*, 2.

[53] Schwarzenegger, A. (2012). *Total Recall: My Unbelievably True Life Story*. New York: Simon and Schuster.

What are you waiting for? Go for it!

www.ingramcontent.com/pod-product-compliance
Lightning Source LLC
Chambersburg PA
CBHW070654250726

48662CB00001B/115

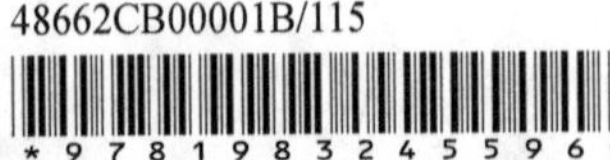